The Renal System
at a Glance

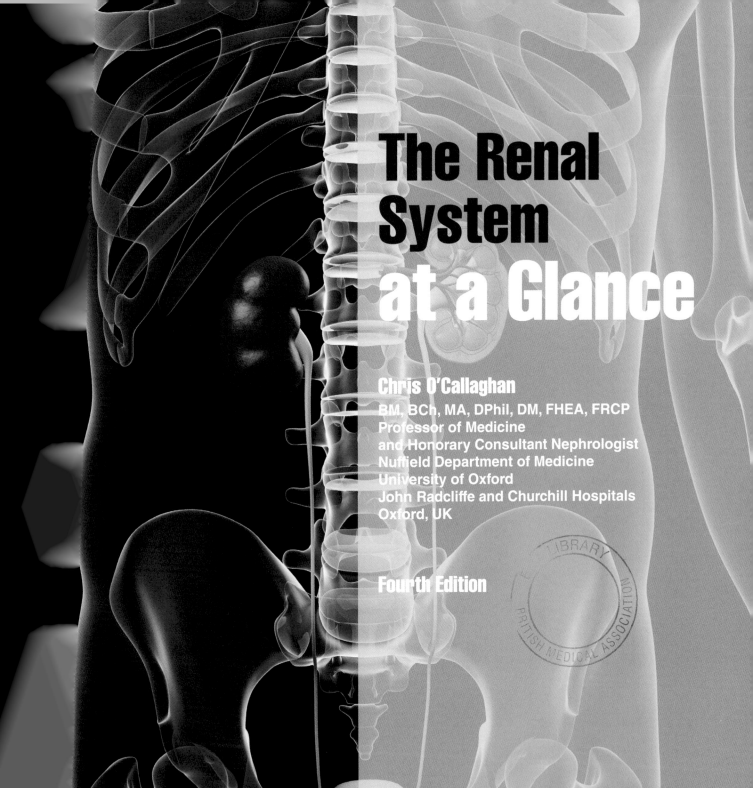

The Renal System
at a Glance

Chris O'Callaghan

BM, BCh, MA, DPhil, DM, FHEA, FRCP
Professor of Medicine
and Honorary Consultant Nephrologist
Nuffield Department of Medicine
University of Oxford
John Radcliffe and Churchill Hospitals
Oxford, UK

Fourth Edition

WILEY Blackwell

This edition first published 2017 © 2017 by John Wiley & Sons, Ltd.

Registered office: John Wiley & Sons, Ltd, The Atrium, Southern Gate, Chichester, West Sussex, PO19 8SQ, UK

Editorial offices: 9600 Garsington Road, Oxford, OX4 2DQ, UK
The Atrium, Southern Gate, Chichester, West Sussex, PO19 8SQ, UK
350 Main Street, Malden, MA 02148-5020, USA

For details of our global editorial offices, for customer services and for information about how to apply for permission to reuse the copyright material in this book please see our website at www.wiley.com/wiley-blackwell

Library of Congress Cataloging-in-Publication Data

Names: O'Callaghan, C. A., author.
Title: The renal system at a glance / C. A. O'Callaghan.
Other titles: At a glance series (Oxford, England)
Description: 4th edition. | Chichester, West Sussex: John Wiley
    & Sons, Ltd., 2017. | Series: At a glance series | Includes index.
Identifiers: LCCN 2016011606 (print) | LCCN 2016012471 (ebook) | ISBN
    9781118393871 (pbk.) | ISBN 9781118393857 (pdf) | ISBN 9781118393864 (epub)
Subjects: | MESH: Kidney–physiology | Kidney–physiopathology | Kidney Diseases
Classification: LCC RC902 (print) | LCC RC902 (ebook) | NLM WJ 301 | DDC
    616.6/1—dc23
LC record available at https://lccn.loc.gov/2016011606

A catalogue record for this book is available from the British Library.

Wiley also publishes its books in a variety of electronic formats. Some content that appears in print may not be available in electronic books.

Cover image: ©gettyimages/SCIEPRO

Set in Minion Pro 9.5/11.5 by Aptara
Printed and bound in Singapore by Markono Print Media Pte Ltd

1   2017

Contents

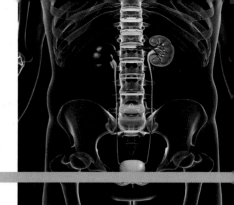

Preface to the fourth edition vii
Introduction and how to use this book ix
Abbreviations x
Glossary xii
Nomenclature xiv
Normal values xv
About the companion website xvii

Part 1 **Introduction** **1**
1 The kidney: structural overview 2
2 The kidney: functional overview 4
3 Development of the renal system 6
4 Clinical features of kidney disease 8
5 The kidney: laboratory investigations and diagnostic imaging 10

Part 2 **Filtration and blood flow** **13**
6 Renal vascular biology 14
7 Glomerular filtration 16
8 Renal vascular disease 18
9 Erythropoietin and anemia in renal disease 20

Part 3 **Sodium and water** **23**
10 Renal sodium handling 24
11 The kidney and water handling 26
12 Regulation of body sodium and body water 28
13 Disorders of sodium and water metabolism 30
14 Hyponatremia and hypernatremia 32
15 The edema states: sodium and water retention 34

Part 4 **Potassium** **37**
16 Renal potassium handling 38
17 Regulation of potassium metabolism 40
18 Hypokalemia and hyperkalemia 42

Part 5 **Acid-base** **45**
19 Renal acid-base and buffer concepts 46
20 Renal acid-base handling 48
21 Acid-base regulation and responses to acid-base disturbances 50
22 Clinical disorders of acid-base metabolism and metabolic acidosis 52
23 Metabolic alkalosis, respiratory acidosis, and respiratory alkalosis 54
24 Renal tubular acidosis 56

Part 6 **Divalent ions – calcium, phosphate and magnesium** **59**
25 Calcium, phosphate, and magnesium metabolism 60
26 Regulation of divalent ions and disorders of phosphate and magnesium 62
27 Hypocalcemia and hypercalcemia 64

Part 7 **Drugs and genetic disorders** **67**
28 Drug and organic molecule handling by the kidney 68
29 Renal pharmacology: diuretics 70
30 Hereditary disorders of tubular transport 72
31 Polycystic kidney disease 74

Part 8 **Glomerular and tubulointerstitial disease** **77**
32 Glomerular disease: an overview 78
33 Glomerular pathologies and their associated diseases 80
34 Specific diseases affecting the glomeruli 82
35 Proteinuria and the nephrotic syndrome 84
36 Tubulointerstitial disease 86

Part 9 **Systemic conditions and the renal system** **89**
37 Hypertension: causes and clinical evaluation 90
38 Hypertension: complications and therapy 92
39 Pregnancy and the renal system 94
40 Diabetes mellitus and the kidney 96

Part 10 **Acute kidney injury and chronic kidney disease** **99**
41 Acute kidney injury: pathophysiology 100
42 Acute kidney injury: clinical aspects 102
43 Chronic kidney disease and kidney function in the elderly 104
44 Severe chronic kidney disease and renal bone disease 106
45 Severe chronic kidney disease: clinical complications and their management 108
46 Treatment of kidney failure with dialysis 110
47 Peritoneal dialysis and continuous hemofiltration 112
48 Renal transplantation 114
49 Global kidney medicine 116

Part 11 **Stones, infection and cancer** **119**
50 Urinary tract infection 120
51 Urinary tract stones 122
52 Urinary tract cancer 124

Case studies and questions 126
Answers 129
Index 133

Preface to the fourth edition

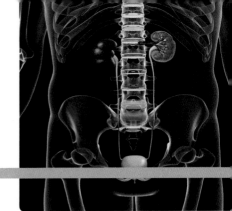

The aim of the first edition of this book (*The Kidney at a Glance*) was to provide a concise and up-to-date account of the renal system in health and disease. Since that edition in 2000, there have been many exciting new developments in our understanding of the kidney, renal and urinary system, and diseases affecting them, and this edition has been completely revised to incorporate these developments. The content has also been reorganized to integrate the basic science and clinical material in a way that should be useful for all curricula, including problem-based learning. Chapters are grouped in sections that provide an integrated account of each topic from basic science to clinical disorders.

New developments include the role of new ion channels, transporters, and associated molecules, such as barttin, the role of glomerular slit pore proteins such as nephrin and podocin in proteinuria, the function of the polycystin complex in polycystic kidney diseases, the role of WNK kinases in hyperkalemic hypertension, FGF23 in renal phosphate excretion, and the role of flow-activated BK potassium channels in the kidney. In addition, new drugs and therapies are available such as direct renin inhibitors, calcimimetics, phosphate-binding resins, and new approaches to immunosuppression. The latest guidance and approaches to acute kidney injury, chronic kidney disease,

and renal replacement therapy have been incorporated where appropriate. There are also new chapters on glomerular filtration and on global kidney medicine. The nomenclature and abbreviations for ion channels, genes, molecules, diseases, and other terms have been completely updated throughout.

This book aims to synthesize all this new information and make sense of it. The book is principally aimed at students, but as with previous editions, it should also be useful to doctors, nurses, or other healthcare professionals who wish to learn about or update themselves on the kidney and renal system in health and disease. This approach has proved very popular, and the book has been circulated worldwide and has been translated into various languages including Chinese, Japanese, Russian, Indonesian, and Greek. Feedback from many readers of the previous editions has guided the writing of this edition and I am grateful to all those who have written to me with their comments. I am grateful to Professor Ian Roberts, Dr. John Scoble, and Dr. Anil Chalisey for permission to use their images in Chapters 7, 51, and 31, respectively. I am also especially grateful for the support and advice of Professor Barry Brenner of Harvard University who coauthored the first edition with me and to many other fine colleagues who have taught me about the renal system over the years.

Chris O'Callaghan

Preface to the first edition

The last few years have seen huge advances in our understanding of how the kidney works and how abnormalities of renal function can affect the whole body. These developments have often resulted from the application of molecular biology, which has led to the cloning of the major transport molecules, channels, and receptors in the kidney, and from careful physiologic studies of the function of these molecules in health and disease. These advances in basic science have transformed the field into one that is highly rational and understandable at all levels from molecular studies of the transporter proteins to clinical studies of patients. As an example, although drugs such as loop diuretics have been prescribed for many years, we now know the precise transporter molecules, which they inhibit, and we can now teach, study, and understand their actions on patients in a completely rational manner. Unfortunately, much of this new information has remained in specialist journals in a piecemeal fashion that makes it difficult for students or physicians to access or put into context.

Our intention is to bring this science in a clear manner to all who need to understand it. We believe that all medical students, doctors, and other health-care providers need to understand the kidney, which is the site of action of so many commonly prescribed drugs and plays a key role in the pathophysiology of so many common disorders, including congestive heart failure and hypertension. We have written this book to draw all this new information together and integrate it with the traditional concepts of renal function and disease. We hope that this new approach, which integrates all the relevant disciplines, including molecular biology, physiology, and clinical medicine, will be of use to all whose work involves the actions of the kidney. We believe that this applies to all students of medicine and all physicians. We also hope that this book will provide the information necessary for others, such as nurses, or nonclinical scientists to rapidly familiarize themselves with the parts of the subject which they need to know.

We have particularly emphasized an understanding of the normal mechanisms and the pathophysiology of the renal system. Although new drugs and treatments may be developed, they must act on the same systems and the same diseases, so knowledge of basic renal function and pathophysiology will stand the reader in good stead for many years to come. This is an exciting field and to do it justice, we have set up a companion website, which will provide a range of supplementary information, including self-assessment material and keypoint summaries. Do please visit the site at *www.ataglanceseries.com/renalsystem*.

We are very grateful to our publishers for their enthusiasm and support; without them, this work would not have been possible. Lastly, we would like to thank our families for their support and all those who have kindly commented on the manuscript, especially Dr. C.G. Winearls, Dr. J.D. Firth, and Dr. R.M. Hilton. Their advice has been extremely helpful, and any deficiencies that remain are entirely our own.

Chris O'Callaghan
Barry M. Brenner

Introduction and how to use this book

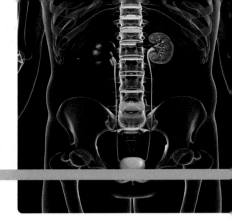

This book provides a comprehensive course in the major aspects of renal and urinary system science and disease, which is suitable for students of medicine and other life sciences. It should also be a valuable learning and revision tool for those in more advanced training and a handy reference book for more experienced clinicians. In particular, the incorporation of the very latest molecular renal physiology makes this book ideal for those familiar with traditional renal science to update themselves with this new information. Other healthcare workers, especially nurses and pharmacists, may find the book helpful too.

Although most doctors are not renal physicians, the kidney is involved in many conditions. Almost all doctors prescribe drugs that act on the kidney, such as diuretics, on a regular basis, and are involved in assessing and adjusting fluid and electrolyte balance. It is now recognized that around 5–10% of the population have chronic kidney disease. For this reason, a clear understanding of renal science is essential for all who care for patients, and this book should provide the basis for such an understanding. As well as detailing specific renal diseases, there is full coverage of the major fluid and electrolyte disturbances.

A strong emphasis has been placed on explaining the mechanisms of disease because, unlike drugs or even clinical investigations, the mechanisms of a disease will be the same throughout a clinician's career. A good understanding of renal and electrolyte abnormalities will last a professional lifetime.

Renal science has undergone dramatic transformations over recent years, especially with the molecular understanding of the major transporters and ion channels, and this makes the whole subject much easier to understand. We now know the precise molecular mechanisms of action of key drugs, such as furosemide and the other diuretics, and it is now possible to give a clear explanation of their precise actions in a way that was not previously possible.

The individual chapters are arranged so that the essential material is encapsulated in the pictures, and in general, it will not be necessary to try to memorize material that is not in the pictures. The text provides an explanation of the subject to accompany the pictures. Reading a rational explanation of the subject matter should make it easy to understand the material and subsequently to use the pictures as quick revision aids. Generally, if a subject is not understood properly, it is very difficult to learn, and the text should help learning by providing a rational explanation of all that is presented. Some readers find it helpful to add their own annotations to the pictures when studying or revising.

Several topics have been included for completeness and for more advanced readers, such as those training in internal medicine, pediatrics, and nephrology, or those aiming for particularly high marks in their examinations. A good example would be renal tubular acidosis. Recommended international nonproprietary names (rINNs) have been used for drugs throughout the text, but older commonly used names are also given.

Diagrams

The diagrams of ion movement are all drawn in the same style. In each case, the yellow left side of the image and, therefore, of the cell, is the tubular lumen, and the blue right side of the image and, therefore, of the cell, is the renal interstitium which leads on to the blood. The Na^+/K^+ ATPase is always shown in yellow. In addition, other transporter molecules are drawn as pink circles if they mediate active transport or as blue circles if they mediate passive transport. Ion channels are shown as two straight lines (see Chapter 2).

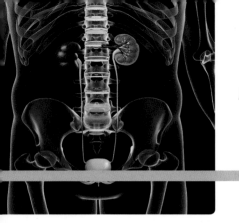

Abbreviations

ACE	angiotensin-converting enzyme
ACEI	angiotensin-converting enzyme inhibitor
ACR	albumin:creatinine ratio
ADH	antidiuretic hormone or vasopressin
ADPKD	autosomal dominant polycystic kidney disease
AE1	anion exchanger 1
AGBM	antiglomerular basement membrane antibody
AKI	acute kidney injury
ANA	antinuclear antibody
ANCA	antineutrophil cytoplasmic antibody
AngII	angiotensin II
ANP	atrial natriuretic peptide
AQP	aquaporin
ARB	angiotensin II receptor blocker
ARPKD	autosomal recessive polycystic kidney disease
ASOT/ASLO	anti-streptolysin O titre
AT1	type 1 angiotensin II receptor
ATN	acute tubular necrosis
ATP	adenosine triphosphate
AVP	vasopressin (ADH)
BJP	Bence Jones protein
BK	big potassium channel = maxi K channel
BNP	brain natriuretic peptide
BP	blood pressure
BUN	blood urea nitrogen
C3	a component of the common complement cascade, lowered by both classic and alternative complement activation
C4	a component of the alternative complement cascade
CA	carbonic anhydrase
cAMP	cyclic adenosine monophosphate
CaR	calcium-sensing receptor = CaSR
CD2	protein number 2 in the CD (cluster of differentiation) classification
CD25	interleukin 2 receptor alpha chain
CD2AP	CD2-associated protein
cGMP	cyclic guanosine monophosphate
CKD	chronic kidney disease
CKD-EPI	Chronic Kidney Disease Epidemiology Collaboration
CNP	C-type natriuretic peptide
CRP	C-reactive protein

CT/CAT	computed tomography
DCT	distal convoluted tubule
DMSA	dimercaptosuccinic acid—used for radionuclide studies of renal function
dsDNA	double-stranded DNA
DTPA	diethylenetriaminepenta-acetic acid—used for radionuclide studies of renal perfusion
ECaC1	epithelial calcium channel 1 = TRPV5
ECG/EKG	electrocardiography
EDTA	ethylenediaminetetra-acetic acid
ENaC	epithelial sodium channel—amiloride sensitive
EPO	erythropoietin
EpoR	erythropoietin receptor
ESR	erythrocyte sedimentation rate
FF	filtration fraction
FGF23	fibroblast growth factor 23 (despite its name FGF23 is not a fibroblast growth factor)
FIH1	factor inhibiting HIF1α
FK506	tacrolimus
FKBP	FK506 (tacrolimus) binding protein
FMD	fibromuscular dysplasia
GBM	glomerular basement membrane
GDNF	glial-derived neurotrophic factor
GFR	glomerular filtration rate
HIF1α	hypoxia-inducible factor 1 alpha
HIVAN	HIV-associated nephropathy
JGA	juxtaglomerular apparatus
KCC	potassium chloride co-transporter
MAG3	mercaptoacetyl-triglycine
MDR1	multidrug resistance ATPase
MR/MRI	magnetic resonance imaging
NaDC3	sodium dicarboxylate co-transporter 3
NBC	sodium bicarbonate co-transporter
NCC	sodium chloride co-transporter—thiazide sensitive
NCX	sodium calcium exchanger
NHE3	sodium/hydrogen (Na^+/H^+) exchanger 3
NKCC2	sodium potassium chloride co-transporter channel 2—furosemide sensitive
NO	nitric oxide
NPR-A	natriuretic peptide receptor A
NPs	natriuretic peptides
NPT2	sodium phosphate co-transporter 2

NSAIDs	nonsteroidal anti-inflammatory drugs
OAT	organic anion transporter
OCT	organic cation transporter
PAH	*p*-aminohippuric acid
PCT	proximal convoluted tubule
PGE2	prostaglandin E2
PGI2	prostaglandin I2
pH	negative logarithm of the hydrogen ion concentration
PHD	prolyl hydroxylase domain enzyme
p*Ka*	the dissociation constant for an acid-base couple
PKD	polycystic kidney disease
PMCA	plasma membrane Ca^{2+} ATPase
PSA	prostate-specific antigen
PTH	parathyroid hormone
pVHL	von Hippel–Lindau tumor suppressor protein
RAS	renal artery stenosis
RBF	renal blood flow
ROMK	renal outer medullary potassium channel
RPF	renal plasma flow
RTA	renal tubular acidosis
RVH	renovascular hypertension
SEP	sclerosing encapsulating peritonitis
SGLT2	sodium glucose transporter 2
SLE	systemic lupus erythematosus
TAL	thick ascending loop of Henle
TRPM6	epithelial magnesium channel
TRPV5	epithelial calcium channel, previously called ECaC1
UMOD	uromodulin
URAT1	urate transporter
UT-A1	urea transporter A1
VMA	vanillylmandelic acid

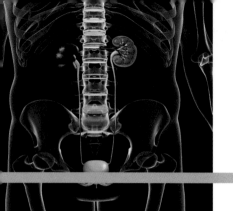

Glossary

Active transport   A transport process requiring energy in the form of ATP.

Aldosterone   A steroid produced by the adrenal cortex promoting sodium reabsorption in the collecting ducts.

Angiotensin II   A protein that is a potent vasoconstrictor; it acts via aldosterone and directly on the nephron to promote salt retention.

Antidiuretic hormone (ADH or vasopressin)   See Vasopressin.

Antiport   The same as counter-transport.

Anuria   The complete absence of urine.

Apoptosis   Programmed cell death.

Atrial natriuretic peptide (ANP)   A peptide produced by cardiac cells causing enhanced sodium excretion.

Bence Jones protein (BJP)   Antibody light chains produced by B-cell dysplasias such as myeloma, which are present in the urine and may cause renal disease.

Bowman's capsule   The tubular epithelial component of the glomerulus, which envelops the glomerular capillaries to form a space, Bowman's space, into which the filtrate passes.

Calyces   Divisions of the renal pelvis. The major calyces split into minor calyces and the renal papillae project into the minor calyces.

Carbonic anhydrase   An enzyme catalyzing the reaction of carbon dioxide and water.

Casts   Cylindrical aggregates of cells or protein debris formed in the distal tubules or collecting ducts.

Cloaca   The primitive excretory region in the fetus shared by both the urinary and gut drainage systems.

Collagen   A key protein in connective tissue.

Complement   A series of proteins triggered by infection or inflammation which promote tissue inflammation and destruction. C4 is a component of the alternative complement cascade. C3 is a component of the common complement cascade, lowered by both classic and alternative complement activation.

Cortex   The outer renal tissue containing the glomeruli and most of the proximal and distal tubules.

Co-transport   Transport of two molecules or ions in the same direction.

Counter-transport   Transport of two molecules or ions in opposite directions.

Creatine kinase   An enzyme released from damaged muscle.

Creatinine   A metabolic product of creatine metabolism filtered and secreted by the kidney.

Cytokines   Soluble molecules that can alter cellular behavior and attributes, particularly during inflammatory processes.

Doppler studies   Clinical studies that measure flow in vessels by the Doppler effect on ultrasound waves.

Efficacy   The effectiveness of treatment.

End-stage renal disease   A loss of renal function so severe that life cannot be maintained without renal replacement therapy.

Erythropoietin   A protein produced in the kidney that promotes red blood cell formation.

Filtration fraction   This is the ratio GFR/RPF and is a measure of the proportion of plasma passing through the glomerular capillaries that is filtered.

Fundoscopy   Looking at the retina, usually with an ophthalmoscope.

Glomerulonephritis   Disease of the glomeruli, usually with inflammation.

Hematocrit   The proportion of the blood that is made up of red blood cells.

Hematuria   Blood in the urine. Frank hematuria means visible blood in the urine.

Homeostasis   The maintenance of normal body conditions.

Hydrostatic pressure   The physical pressure of water---equivalent to hydraulic pressure.

Immunostaining, immunoperoxidase, immunofluorescence   Histological methods using synthetically labeled antibodies to detect the presence of proteins or natural antibodies in tissue specimens.

Interstitial cells   Renal cells that support the matrix of the kidney but are not part of the nephron.

Interstitium   Connective tissue; in the kidney, the tissue that is not composed of vessels, nephrons, ducts, or other specialized components.

Inulin   A substance freely filtered but neither reabsorbed nor secreted, which can be used to estimate glomerular filtration rate.

Iso-osmotic   A process that occurs without causing a change in osmolality. Iso-osmotic reabsorption of sodium from the filtrate means that the sodium brings water with it, so that there is no overall change in the osmolality of the filtrate.

Juxtaglomerular apparatus (JGA)   The combination of the tubular cells of the macula densa, granular afferent arteriolar cells that secrete renin, and extraglomerular mesangial cells.

Lateral   Away from the midline. Medial is toward the midline.

Macula densa   A patch of columnar tubular epithelial cells that forms part of the JGA and may sense tubular ion concentration. It is situated at the junction of the thick ascending limb of the loop of Henle and the early distal tubule.

Medial   Toward the midline. Lateral is away from the midline.

Medulla   The inner kidney constituting the renal pyramids and containing the loops of Henle, the medullary and papillary collecting ducts, and the vasa recta.

Mesangial cells   Renal cells in the glomerulus that support the glomerular capillary walls and may have some contractile function.

Mesonephric duct   The duct that forms the ejaculatory duct in men.

Mesonephros   The second fetal kidney.

Metanephros   The final fetal kidney which forms the adult kidney.

Myoglobin   A muscle protein with oxygen-binding capacity, which is toxic to renal tubules.

Myoglobinuria   Myoglobin in urine.

Nephrin   A major filtration slit pore protein.

Nephritic syndrome   Acute glomerulonephritis with hypertension, renal impairment, and often edema.

Nephrocalcinosis   The diffuse deposition of calcium in the renal tissue.

Nephrolithiasis   The formation of renal stones.

Nephron   The basic excretory unit consisting of the glomerulus and its tubules.

Nephrotic syndrome Proteinuria sufficient to cause a low serum albumin and peripheral edema.

Oncotic pressure Colloid osmotic pressure.

Ontogeny The pathway of cell differentiation.

Osmolality The concentration of solutes in a given weight of water.

Osmosis The movement of water through a semipermeable membrane from a solution of low osmotic strength (low concentration) to one of high osmotic strength (high concentration).

Ostial lesion Lesion at the opening of a vessel.

PAH *p*-Aminohippurate: a substance completely cleared by a single pass through the kidney, which can be used to estimate renal blood flow.

Papillary ducts Ducts into which collecting ducts drain and which open out at the tip of the renal papilla into a minor calyx.

Paracellular Around the side of cells.

Paramesonephric duct The duct that forms the female reproductive tract.

Paraprotein A protein that is present at high concentrations and is usually an antibody produced by a B-cell dysplasia, such as myeloma.

Parathyroid hormone A protein produced by the parathyroid gland; it acts on the kidney to promote phosphate excretion, calcium reabsorption, and vitamin D production, and it promotes calcium and phosphate release from bone.

Paresthesia Tingling numbness in the extremities.

Passive transport A transport process that does not require energy.

Podocalyxin A negatively charged glycoprotein that covers the pores in the glomerular capillary endothelial cells and forms part of the glomerular basement membrane.

Podocin A filtration slit pore protein.

Podocytes The thin tubular epithelial cells which form part of the glomerular filtration barrier and cover the urinary aspect of the glomerular capillaries.

Polycythemia Excess red blood cells in the blood.

Polydipsia Excess water intake.

Polyuria Excess urine volume.

Pontine myelinolysis Destruction of neural tissue in the pons when there is rapid correction of disordered osmolality.

Pronephros The earliest fetal kidney which is nonfunctional.

Renal hilus The medial aspect of the kidney containing the entrance sites of the renal artery and vein and the renal pelvis.

Renal pelvis The upper portion of the ureter leading into the calyces.

Renal replacement therapy Treatment that takes over the function of the kidneys, usually dialysis, hemofiltration, or transplantation.

Renin An enzyme released by the JGA, which results in the formation of angiotensin II.

Reticulocyte A nucleated red blood cell precursor.

Rhabdomyolysis Muscle damage or destruction causing the release of nephrotoxic myoglobin.

Slit diaphragm The tight junctions between adjacent podocytes which form part of the glomerular filtration barrier.

Tamm–Horsfall protein Encoded by the UMOD gene. A protein secreted by tubular cells, especially in the thick ascending limb of the loop of Henle. It helps to hold together casts which can form in the tubules.

Transepithelial gradient An electrical or concentration gradient across the tubular epithelium.

Urea A waste product of protein catabolism made by the liver and filtered and reabsorbed by the kidney.

Uricosuric Causing uric acid excretion in the urine.

Uroplakin Protein lining urinary epithelium, which forms a barrier between the cell and urine.

Vasa recta Paired descending and ascending blood vessels, which travel from the cortex to the medulla and back into the cortex with the loops of Henle.

Vasculitis A disease process causing vessel inflammation and damage.

Vasopressin A polypeptide released by the posterior pituitary gland causing water reabsorption in the collecting duct.

Vesical Relating to the bladder, e.g., ureterovesical.

Vitamin D A steroid hormone metabolized in the kidney to the active form 1,25-dihydroxycholecalciferol, which promotes calcium and phosphate absorption from the gut as a principal action.

Wolffian duct The same as the mesonephric duct.

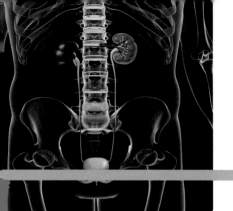

Nomenclature

USA and UK differences in spelling and nomenclature

The main differences relate to the use of "ae" in the UK and "e" in the USA.

USA	UK
anemia	anaemia
diarrhea	diarrhoea
edema	oedema
fetal	foetal
hematocrit	haematocrit
hemoglobin	haemoglobin
hypercalcemia	hypercalcaemia
hyperkalemia	hyperkalaemia
hypernatremia	hypernatraemia
hyponatremia	hyponatraemia
paresthesia	paraesthesia
polycythemia	polycythaemia

In the USA, conventional units such as mg/dL are used, whereas in Europe and most other countries, the SI (Système International) units such as mmol/L are used. For creatinine, to convert from mmol/L to mg/dL, divide by 88.4.

A number of terms differ, in particular:

USA	UK
cyclo porine	ciclosporin
epinephrine	adrenaline (although in the UK epinephrine is increasingly used)
furosemide	frusemide
vasopressin	antidiuretic hormone (ADH)

Normal values

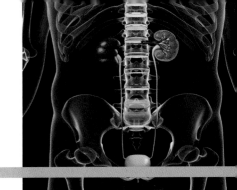

Table 1 Blood biochemistry

Basic electrolytes

Sodium	135–145 mmol/L	135–145 mEq/L
Potassium	3.5–5.0 mmol/L	3.5–5.0 mEq/L
Urea	2.5–8.0 mmol/L	BUN 7–22 mg/dL
Creatinine	60–130 µmol/L	0.7–1.5 mg/dL
Chloride	90–105 mmol/L	90–105 mEq/L
Bicarbonate (venous)	22–28 mmol/L	22–28 mEq/L
Anion gap $(Na^+ + K^+) - (HCO_3^- + Cl^-)$	12–16 mmol/L	12–16 mEq/L
Plasma osmolality	275–295 mmol/kg	275–295 mOsm/kg

Bone

Total protein	60–80 g/L	6.0–8.0 g/dL
Albumin	35–50 g/L	3.5–5.0 g/dL
Calcium	2.15–2.55 mmol/L	8.6–10.2 mg/dL
Ionized calcium	1.0–1.25 mmol/L	4.0–5.0 mg/dL
Phosphate	0.8–1.5 mmol/L	2.5–4.6 mg/dL
Magnesium	0.8–1.2 mmol/L	1.8–3.0 mg/dL
Calcium phosphate product	$3.5–4.2\ mmol^2/L^2$	$43–52\ mg^2/dL^2$

Others

Acid phosphatase	50–115 U/L	
Amylase	25–180 U/L	
Bilirubin	3–17 µmol/L	0.2–1.0 mg/dL
Alkaline phosphatase	80–250 U/L	
Alanine aminotransferase (ALT)	5–40 U/L	
Aspartate aminotransferase (AST)	15–40 U/L	
Gamma-glutamyltransferase (GGT)	10–50 U/L (males) 7–30 U/L (females)	
Creatinine kinase	30–250 U/L (males) 30–180 U/L (females)	
Prostate specific antigen (PSA)	<4.0 µg/L	
Urate	120–420 µmol/L	2.0–7.0 mg/dL

Glucose and lipids

Glucose (random)	3.5–7.8 mmol/L	63–140 mg/dL
Glucose (fasting)	3.5–6.0 mmol/L	63–108 mg/dL
Glycated hemoglobin (glycated HBA_{1C})	<48 mmol/mol	<6.5%
Cholesterol	3.3–7.3 mmol/L	130–280 mg/dL
Ideally	<5.2 mmol/L	<200 mg/dL
HDL cholesterol	0.9–2.0 mmol/L	35–75 mg/dL
Ideally	>1.2 mmol/L	>46 mg/dL
LDL cholesterol	1.5–4.4 mmol/L	38–170 mg/dL
Ideally	<3.4 mmol/L	130 mg/dL
Triglycerides (fasting)	0.6–1.9 mmol/L	53–170 mg/dL

Immunological

C-reactive protein (CRP)	<10 mg/L	<1 mg/dL
Complement C3	0.7–1.7 g/L	70–170 mg/dL
Complement C4	0.15–0.5 g/L	15–50 mg/dL
IgA	0.8–4.0 g/L	80–400 mg/dL
IgG	6–16 g/L	600–1600 mg/dL
IgM	0.5–2.0 g/L	50–200 mg/dL
IgE	<12–240 µg/L	<41 U/L

Table 2 Urine biochemistry

Sodium	100–300 mmol/24 h	100–300 mEq/24 h
Calcium	2.5–7.5 mmol/24 h	10–30 mg/24 h
Protein	<0.1 g/24 h	<100 mg/24 h
Creatinine	10–18 mmol/24 h	1.1–2.0 mg/24 h
Creatinine clearance	80–140 mL/min	
Urine osmolality	60–1200 mmol/kg	500–1200 mOsm/kg

Proteinuria

Approximate equivalent values. ACR—albumin : creatinine ratio, PCR—protein : creatinine ratio. ACR of ≥30 mg/mmol is significant proteinuria. ACR > 2.5 mg/mmol in men or >3.5 mg/mmol in women is significant in diabetic patients

ACR mg/ mmol	PCR mg/ mmol	24 h proteinuria g/24 h	PCR mg/mg or g/g
30	50	0.5	6
70	100	1.0	12

Table 3 Hematology

Hemoglobin	130–170 g/L (males) 120–160 g/L (females)	
White cell count (WBC)	$4.0–11.0 \times 10^9$/L	$4.0–11.0 \times 10^3$/mm^3
Platelets	$150–400 \times 10^9$/L	$150–400 \times 10^3$/mm^3
Erythrocyte sedimentation rate (ESR)	1–10 mm/h (<50 years) <20 mm/h (>50 years)	
Plasma viscosity	1.1–1.35 mPa·s	
Prothrombin time (PT)	12–16 s	
International normalized ratio (INR)	1.0–1.3	
Activated partial thromboplastin time (APTT)	21–33 s	
Ferritin	6–110 µg/L (females) 20–260 µg/L (males)	6–110 ng/mL 20–260 ng/mL
Vitamin B_{12}	150–700 ng/L	150–700 ng/mL
Red cell folate	100–600 µg/L	100–600 ng/mL

Normal values (*continued*)

Table 4 Arterial blood gases

PaO_2	10.6–14.5 kPa	80–110 mm Hg
$PaCO_2$	4.0–6.0 kPa	30–45 mm Hg
pH	7.35–7.45	
H^+	35–45 nmol/L	
Bicarbonate (arterial)	19–24 mmol/L	19–24 mEq/L

Table 5 Chronic kidney disease and eGFR (see Chapter 43, page 104)

Stage	eGFR (mL/min/1.73 m^2)
G1	≥90 + kidney abnormality
G2	60–89 + kidney abnormality
G3a	45–59
G3b	30–44
G4	15–29
G5	<15

The urine albumin:creatinine ratio in mg/mmol provides the "A" staging (A1 if < 3, A2 if 3–30 and A3 if >30 mg/mmol).

About the companion website

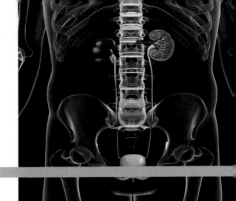

Don't forget to visit the companion website for this book:

www.ataglanceseries.com/renalsystem

There you will find valuable material
designed to enhance your learning, including:

- Interactive multiple-choice questions
- Chapter key points for revision
- Study guide
- Flashcards of key figures with interactive on/off
  labels
- Animations

Scan this QR code to visit the companion website

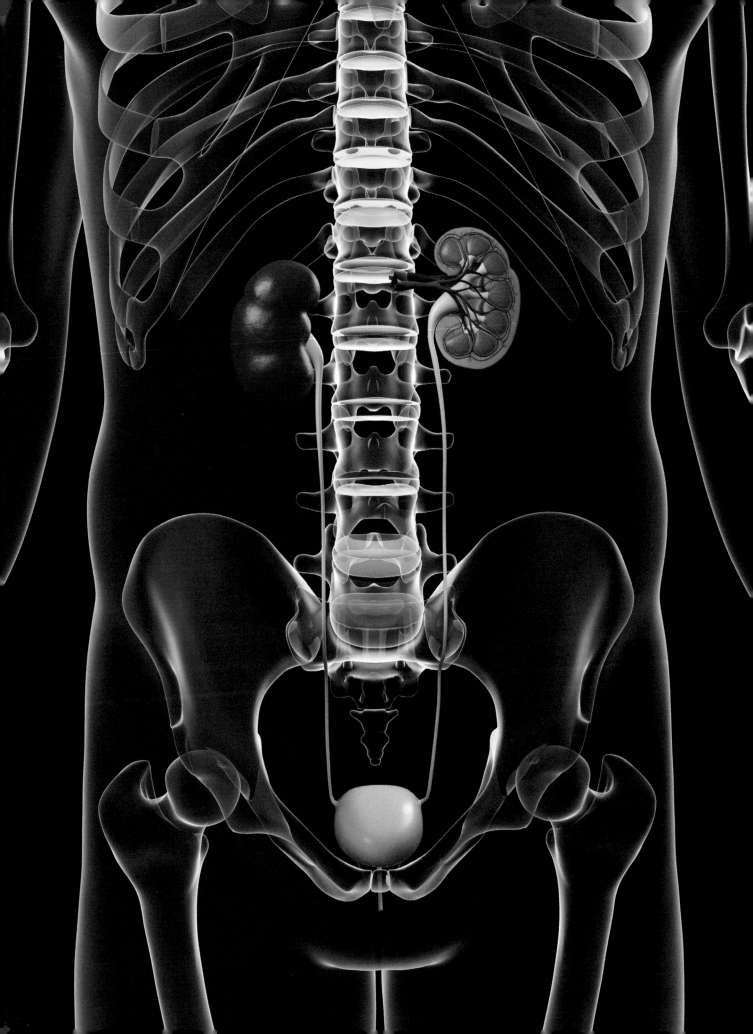

Introduction

Part 1

Chapters

1   The kidney: structural overview   2
2   The kidney: functional overview   4
3   Development of the renal system   6
4   Clinical features of kidney disease   8
5   The kidney: laboratory investigations and diagnostic imaging   10

Don't forget to visit the companion website for this book
www.ataglanceseries.com/renalsystem

1 The kidney: structural overview

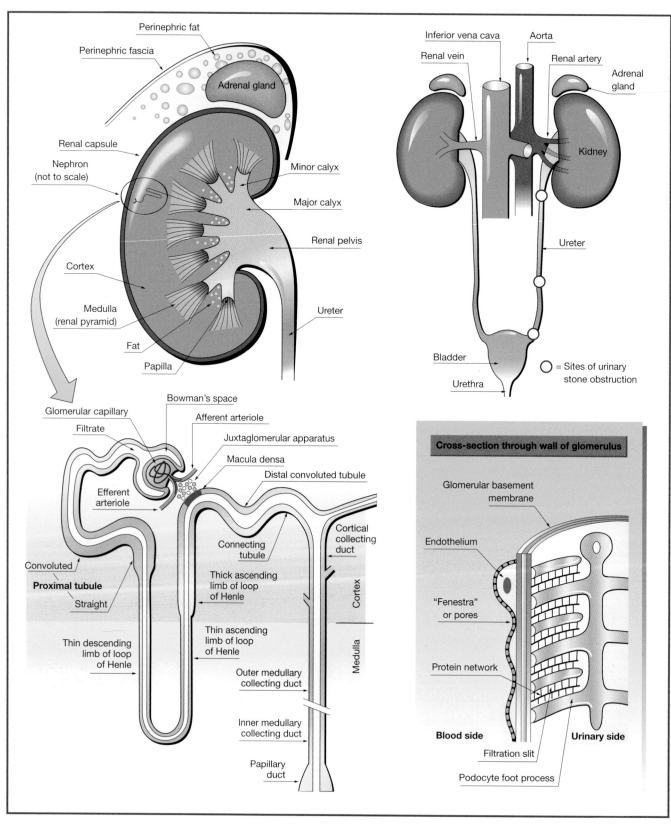

The Renal System at a Glance, Fourth Edition. Chris O'Callaghan. © 2017 John Wiley & Sons, Ltd. Published 2017 by John Wiley & Sons, Ltd.
Companion website: www.ataglanceseries.com/renalsystem

Gross anatomy

The kidney

The kidneys lie behind the peritoneum at the back of the abdominal cavity, extending from the twelfth thoracic vertebra (T12) to the third lumbar vertebra (L3). The right kidney is lower than the left because of the presence of the liver. During inspiration, both kidneys are pushed down as the diaphragm contracts. Each kidney is covered by a fibrous capsule. This is further surrounded by perinephric fat and then by the perinephric (perirenal) fascia, which also enclose the adrenal gland. The renal cortex is the outer zone of the kidney and the renal medulla is the inner zone made up of the renal pyramids. The cortex contains all the glomeruli, and the medulla contains the loops of Henle, the vasa recta, and the final portions of the collecting ducts.

Vessels and nerves

Blood vessels and the ureter connect with the kidney at the renal hilus. The renal artery arises from the aorta and usually divides into three branches. Two pass in front of the ureter and one goes behind it. Five or six small veins come together to form the renal vein, which leaves the kidney in front of the anterior branch of the renal artery and enters the inferior vena cava. The position of the lymphatics and the renal sympathetic nerves is variable. The lymphatics drain to the lateral aortic lymph nodes. Sympathetic nerves supply the renal vasculature and juxtaglomerular apparatus, and to a lesser extent the rest of the nephron. Afferent fibers enter the spinal cord at T10, T11, and T12.

The draining system for urine

Within the kidney, the pelvis of the ureter divides into two or three major calyces, each of which subdivides into two or three minor calyces. Each minor calyx contains a renal papilla, which is the apex of a medullary pyramid. The ureter passes out of the kidney behind the peritoneum on the psoas muscle and then enters the pelvis in front of the sacroiliac joint. It moves down the lateral pelvic wall toward the ischial spine and then turns forward and medially to enter the bladder. It passes through the bladder wall for 2 cm before opening into the bladder. Urine passes along the ureter by peristalsis. The ureter has three constrictions where kidney stones can become lodged (see Chapter 51). Afferent nerves from the ureter enter the spinal cord at T11, T12, L1, and L2. The bladder is innervated by S3, S4, and S5.

Microanatomy

The nephron

The nephron is the basic unit of the kidney. Each kidney has 400,000–800,000 nephrons, although this number falls with age.

A nephron consists of the glomerulus and the associated tubule that leads to the collecting duct. Urine is formed by filtration in the glomerulus; it is then modified in the tubules by the reabsorption and secretion of substances. Cortical nephrons occur throughout the renal cortex and have short loops of Henle; juxtamedullary nephrons begin near the corticomedullary junction and have long loops of Henle, which descend deep into the medulla and enable them to concentrate urine effectively. Cortical nephrons outnumber juxtamedullary nephrons by 7 : 1.

Interstitial cells in the kidney

The cortex contains two types of interstitial cell: phagocytic and fibroblast-like cells. Erythropoietin is made in the fibroblast-like cells. Three types of medullary interstitial cells have been identified. One type contains lipid droplets, which may provide precursors for synthesis of prostaglandins in the kidneys.

The glomerulus as a filtration barrier
(see Chapter 7)

The glomerulus is a ball of capillaries surrounded by the Bowman's capsule, a hollow capsule of the tubular epithelium into which urine is filtered. The space into which the urine is filtered is known as Bowman's space. The glomerulus also contains mesangial cells, which provide a scaffold to support capillary loops and have contractile and phagocytic properties. Blood enters the glomerular capillaries from an afferent arteriole and leaves through an efferent arteriole, rather than a venule. Vasoconstriction of this efferent arteriole creates a high hydrostatic pressure in the glomerular capillary, forcing water, ions, and small molecules through the filtration barrier into Bowman's space. Whether a substance is filtered depends on both its molecular size and charge. The filtration barrier has three layers, all of which have a negative charge:

1 *Endothelial cells.* The endothelial cells of the glomerular capillary wall are thin, with numerous 70-nm pores filled with negatively charged glycoprotein, mostly podocalyxin.

2 *Glomerular basement membrane.* This specialized capillary basement membrane has three layers and contains negatively charged glycoproteins attached to a three-dimensional framework of collagen and other proteins.

3 *Epithelial cells of Bowman's capsule.* The epithelial cells or podocytes have long projections from which foot processes arise and attach to the urinary side of the glomerular basement membrane. Foot processes from different podocytes interdigitate, leaving filtration slits of 25–65 nm between them. Across these slits, a protein network rich in nephrin protein forms "slit pores." The pores are the key selectivity barrier in the filtration process and prevent the passage of larger molecules such as albumin.

2 The kidney: functional overview

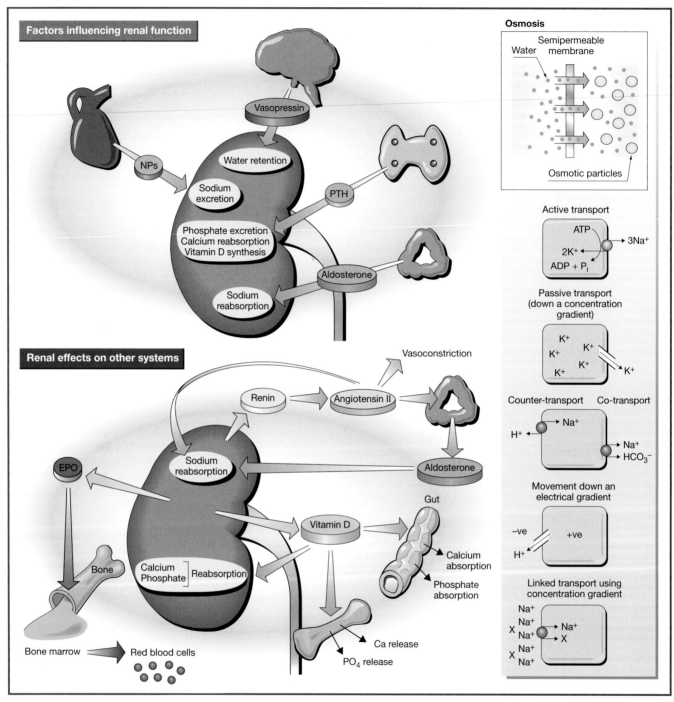

Factors influencing renal function

Osmosis

Renal effects on other systems

The kidney maintains a stable extracellular environment, which supports the function of all body cells. It controls water and ionic balance by regulating the excretion of water, sodium, potassium, chloride, calcium, magnesium, phosphate, and many other substances, and by managing acid-base status.

Tubular function

The urinary filtrate is formed in the glomerulus and flows into the tubules where its volume and content are altered by reabsorption or secretion. Most solute reabsorption occurs in the proximal tubules, and fine adjustments to urine composition are then made in the distal tubule and collecting ducts. The loop of Henle serves to concentrate urine.

The tubular epithelium is only one cell thick. Tubular cells have tight junctions at their apical or luminal edges which separate tubular fluid from peritubular plasma, allowing transport processes to establish concentration gradients across the tubular epithelium. The movement of molecules through these tight junctions is termed "paracellular movement" and is

The Renal System at a Glance, Fourth Edition. Chris O'Callaghan. © 2017 John Wiley & Sons, Ltd. Published 2017 by John Wiley & Sons, Ltd.
Companion website: www.ataglanceseries.com/renalsystem

controlled by the properties of proteins called claudins, which form the main barrier to movement, but can form pores that have size and charge selectivity. In Bowman's capsule, the cells are thin squamous epithelial cells, but in the tubules, the cells are mainly columnar epithelial cells, which are specialized for transport processes.

Proximal tubule

The proximal tubule is initially convoluted and then straightens out as it leads down to the loop of Henle. The tubular cells are tall, columnar epithelial cells with many microvilli, a high surface area, and a well-developed luminal endocytic apparatus. Many substances are actively reabsorbed in the proximal tubule, including sodium, potassium, calcium, phosphate, glucose, amino acids, and water. This reabsorption reduces the volume of filtrate but, because water moves osmotically with the reabsorbed solutes, the filtrate is not concentrated (i.e., iso-osmotic reabsorption). There is also endocytic uptake of filtered proteins by the proximal tubules. Filtered proteins bind to the endocytic receptors megalin and cubilin and are then endocytosed.

Loop of Henle

As the straight proximal tubule becomes the thin descending limb of the loop of Henle, the cells become flatter with fewer microvilli. Next comes the thin ascending limb, followed by the thick ascending limb, which contains predominantly cuboidal cells. The thick ascending limb passes up toward the glomerulus from which it arose, ending at the macula densa (see Chapters 1 and 6).

Juxtaglomerular apparatus

The juxtaglomerular apparatus is a compound structure that consists of three main cell types: a patch of tubular cells termed the **macula densa**, extraglomerular mesangial cells, and granular cells. The granular cells are mainly in the afferent arteriolar wall and secrete renin (see Chapter 6).

Distal tubule

Beyond the macula densa is the distal convoluted tubule. This leads to the collecting tubule, which drains into the collecting duct. The collecting duct has three sections, named according to their depth in the kidney: the cortical collecting duct, the outer medullary collecting duct, and the inner medullary collecting duct. The inner medullary collecting duct flows into a papillary duct, which opens out on a renal papilla into a minor calyx.

Urinary system

The ureters and bladder are lined with epithelial cells. The surface of these cells, which contacts urine, forms a robust permeability barrier and is coated with an organized array of uroplakin molecules. Mutations in these uroplakins are associated with urinary tract malformations.

Blood vessels associated with the loop of Henle

The efferent arterioles in cortical nephrons form a second capillary bed, the peritubular capillaries, which surround the rest of the tubular system. However, in the juxtamedullary nephrons, the efferent arterioles first form vascular bundles that give rise to both the peritubular capillaries and the straight vessels, which in turn form the vasa recta. The descending vasa recta go down into the inner medulla with the loop of Henle. At this level, the vessel branches to form a capillary network, which leads on to the ascending vasa recta. These veins travel upward in close proximity to the descending vasa recta. The vasa recta are the sole blood supply to the medulla (see Chapters 6 and 11).

Transport processes in the tubules

Active transport requires energy expenditure in the form of ATP (e.g., Na^+/K^+ ATPase). Ions or molecules can move by *passive transport* down an electrical or concentration gradient. Water molecules cannot be pumped directly; they move by *osmosis* when there is a concentration gradient of ions or molecules across a semipermeable membrane. If charged particles are moved, electroneutrality is maintained either by *co-transport* in the same direction of a particle of opposite charge or by *counter-transport* in the opposite direction of a particle of the same charge. Molecules can move by *linked transport* to another molecule which is itself moving down an electrical or concentration gradient.

Hormones acting on the kidney

- **Vasopressin (antidiuretic hormone or ADH).** This is a peptide released by the posterior pituitary gland; it promotes water reabsorption in the collecting ducts.
- **Aldosterone.** This is a steroid hormone produced by the adrenal cortex; it promotes sodium reabsorption in the collecting ducts.
- **Natriuretic peptides (NPs).** These are produced mainly by cardiac cells and promote sodium excretion in the collecting ducts.
- **Parathyroid hormone (PTH).** This is a protein produced by the parathyroid gland; it promotes renal phosphate excretion, calcium reabsorption, and vitamin D production.
- **FGF23.** This is produced by bone osteocytes and promotes renal phosphate excretion and inhibits vitamin D production.

Hormones produced by the kidney

- **Renin.** This is a protein released by the juxtaglomerular apparatus; it results in the formation of *angiotensin II*. Angiotensin II acts directly on the proximal tubules and via aldosterone on the distal tubules to promote sodium retention, and is also a potent vasoconstrictor.
- **Vitamin D.** This is a steroid hormone metabolized in the kidney to the active form 1,25-dihydroxycholecalciferol, which promotes calcium and phosphate absorption from the gut as a principal action.
- **Erythropoietin.** This is a protein produced in the kidney; it promotes red blood cell formation in bone marrow.
- **Prostaglandins.** These are produced in the kidney; they have various effects, especially on renal vessel tone.

Development of the renal system

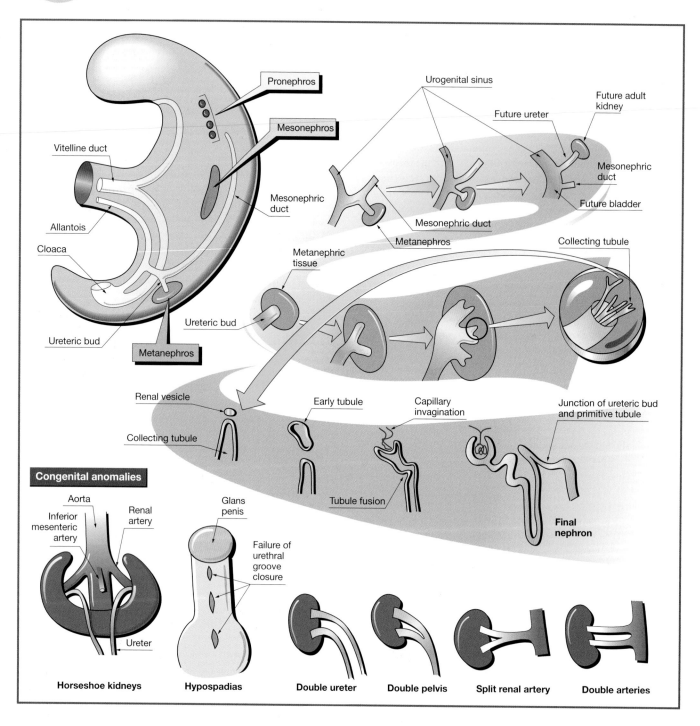

Congenital anomalies

Horseshoe kidneys   Hypospadias   Double ureter   Double pelvis   Split renal artery   Double arteries

The Renal System at a Glance, Fourth Edition. Chris O'Callaghan. © 2017 John Wiley & Sons, Ltd. Published 2017 by John Wiley & Sons, Ltd.
Companion website: www.ataglanceseries.com/renalsystem

The renal and genital systems both develop from the intermediate mesoderm, a collection of cells at the back of the fetal abdominal cavity. Both systems initially drain into the same space, the fetal cloaca. During development, the intermediate mesoderm first forms the pronephros in the cervical region, then the mesonephros below this, and last the metanephros in the pelvic region. The pronephros and mesonephros regress and do not form part of the adult kidney. The metanephros forms the final adult kidney and becomes functional in the second half of pregnancy. Although the fetus swallows amniotic fluid, digests it, and excretes urine into the amniotic fluid, it is the placenta that removes fetal waste products for excretion by the mother's kidneys.

The development of all three kidney systems requires the induction of mesenchyme to become epithelium. In the metanephros, the ureteric bud induces the mesenchyme around its tips to form nephrons. This metanephric mesenchyme forms the tubular system from the glomerulus to the distal nephron, whereas the ureteric bud forms the collecting duct and draining system.

Kidney formation in detail

Around week 4 of gestation, clusters of cells in the intermediate mesoderm form very primitive glomeruli in the cervical region. Together, these form the nonfunctional pronephros which later regresses. However, the lateral portions of the cell cluster at each level fuse to form the mesonephric (or Wolffian) duct, which grows downward and enters the cloaca. As the pronephros regresses, the intermediate mesoderm below it forms the mesonephros. This may function briefly, draining into the mesonephric duct, but it regresses by the end of the second month.

Nephron formation in the metanephros

From week 5 onward, the metanephros forms from intermediate mesoderm cells in the pelvis. Just above the entrance of the mesonephric duct into the cloaca, an outgrowth of the duct called the ureteric bud invades the metanephric tissue mass. The bud dilates to form the renal pelvis, splits progressively to form the calyces, and then small branches elongate to form the collecting tubules. Metanephric tissue at the tips of these collecting ducts aggregates and forms vesicles that develop into tubules. Capillaries invaginate one end of each tubule to form a glomerulus. The newly formed tubule lengthens to form the proximal tubule, loop of Henle, and distal tubule. At the other end, the tubule connects to the collecting tubule that induced its formation.

Renal position and congenital anomalies

In the pelvis, the metanephric kidney receives its blood supply from pelvic branches of the aorta. As the kidneys move upward to their final posterior abdominal position, these original arteries regress and the kidneys are vascularized by the renal arteries, which come off the aorta at a higher level. It is common for some of the earlier arteries to persist as supernumerary renal arteries.

It is also possible for one or both kidneys to remain permanently in the pelvis. If both kidneys stay in the pelvis, they can be forced together and fuse at the lower poles to form a horseshoe kidney, which cannot then rise because of the inferior mesenteric artery above it. If the ureteric bud splits early, the result can be two ureters or two renal pelvises connecting to one ureter.

Bladder and urethra formation

The cloaca is split by a septum into a posterior anorectal region and an anterior urogenital sinus. The ureteric buds form the ureters, which drain into the mesonephric ducts; these then drain into the urogenital sinus. The lower part of the mesonephric ducts becomes absorbed into the wall of the urogenital sinus to form the trigone area of the bladder. This means that, eventually, the mesonephric ducts and the ureters enter the sinus separately. As the kidneys ascend, the openings of the ureters move up the urogenital sinus into the zone that they will occupy when that part of the urogenital sinus becomes the bladder. The lower part of the urogenital sinus forms part of the urethra in both sexes and, in females, it also forms part of the vestibule. In males, the mesonephric ducts form the ejaculatory ducts. A paramesonephric duct also forms and, in females, develops into much of the female upper reproductive tract.

On either side of the anterior cloaca, swellings form into urethral folds, which meet above the cloaca as a genital tubercle. In females, the urethral folds develop into the labia minora. In males, the genital tubercle grows to form a phallus, pulling the urethral folds along to form the lateral walls of a groove below the future glans penis. The folds close over to form the penile urethra. Incomplete fusion of the folds causes hypospadias with a urethral opening along the inferior aspect of the penis. The final distal part of the male urethra is formed by an ingrowth of cells, which form the external urethral meatus.

Molecules implicated in renal development

WT-1, Wilm's tumor gene-1, is a transcription factor expressed at high levels in metanephric mesenchyme (see Chapter 52). In WT-1 knockout mice, no metanephric kidney or gonads form. N-myc, a proto-oncogene, and the transcription factors Pax2 and Pax8, are all expressed in the developing metanephric kidney. Other molecules that may play a role in metanephric development include vascular endothelial growth factor (VEGF), the forkhead transcription factors Foxc1 and Foxc2, the transcription factors Slit2, Robo2, Pod1, and HNF1-beta, the oncogene bcl-2, a secreted glycoprotein Wnt-4, the TGF-β (transforming growth factor-β) family molecules BMP4 and BMP7, the PDGF (platelet-derived growth factor) family proteins, GDNF, and the RET tyrosine kinases. Wnt-4 mutations cause severe renal hypoplasia. Mutations in HNF1-beta cause a syndrome with renal cysts and pancreatic malformations. Abnormalities produced by polycystic kidney disease genes are considered in Chapter 31.

4 Clinical features of kidney disease

History and Examination

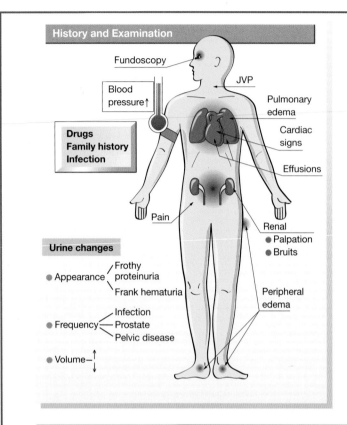

- Fundoscopy
- Blood pressure ↑
- JVP
- Pulmonary edema
- Cardiac signs
- Effusions

Drugs
Family history
Infection

- Pain
- Renal
  - ● Palpation
  - ● Bruits
- Peripheral edema

Urine changes

- ● Appearance — Frothy proteinuria / Frank hematuria
- ● Frequency — Infection / Prostate / Pelvic disease
- ● Volume ↑↓

Examination

Posterior view

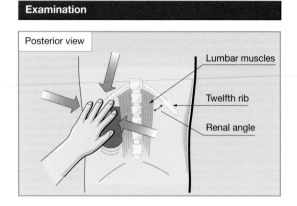

- Lumbar muscles
- Twelfth rib
- Renal angle

Anterior view

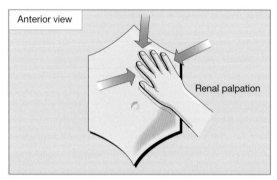

Renal palpation

Urine microscopy

Red cell casts
● Glomerulonephritis

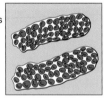

White cell casts

● Inflammation

Infection   Interstitial nephritis

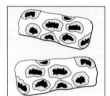

Waxy casts
● Chronic renal disease

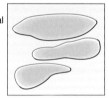

Hyaline casts
● Normal

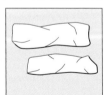

Granular casts
● Normal

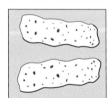

Crystals
● Variable significance

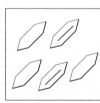

The Renal System at a Glance, Fourth Edition. Chris O'Callaghan. © 2017 John Wiley & Sons, Ltd. Published 2017 by John Wiley & Sons, Ltd.
Companion website: www.ataglanceseries.com/renalsystem

As there are more nephrons in each kidney than are needed to sustain life, significant renal damage can occur without obvious clinical effects. Kidney disease may not become clinically apparent until there is substantial loss of renal function. For this reason, slowly progressing renal diseases can be asymptomatic in the early stages.

History

Pain

Pain is uncommon with renal disease, but can occur if there is urinary obstruction, especially from renal stones. Infection or distention of the renal capsule or of renal cysts, especially in polycystic kidney disease, can also cause pain. Inflammation of the bladder or urethra, usually as a result of infection, can cause dysuria (discomfort on micturition). Rarely, glomerular disease can cause a dull lumbar ache.

Urine appearance and volume

Proteinuria can produce frothy urine and frank *hematuria* is obvious as red or pink urine. Dark urine can also occur with the myoglobinuria of rhabdomyolysis or the hemoglobinuria of hemolysis. Recurrent intermittent frank hematuria suggests immunoglobulin A (IgA) glomerulonephritis in young people or renal tract cancer in elderly people. Glomerular bleeding is present throughout the stream, whereas hematuria only at the beginning of the stream suggests urethral bleeding and hematuria only late in the stream suggests bladder or prostate bleeding.

Increased urinary frequency is an increase in the frequency of micturition. Polyuria is an increase in total urine volume. Increased *urinary frequency*, especially at night, can suggest prostatic enlargement in men or urinary tract infection. *Polyuria* suggests a defect of renal urine-concentrating mechanisms or excess water ingestion. Prostatic enlargement can also cause hesitancy and terminal dribbling as well as obstruction and urinary retention. Total *anuria* is rare and usually suggests urethral or bilateral ureteric obstruction, a severe rapidly progressive glomerulonephritis, or aortic or bilateral renal arterial occlusion.

General history

Always take a full history. Establish whether the patient has a previous history of hypertension, diabetes mellitus, malignancy, or other systemic diseases. Any recent infection, but typically a streptococcal throat infection, can trigger a postinfective glomerulonephritis. The drug history may indicate use of nephrotoxic drugs, especially analgesics or nonsteroidal anti-inflammatory drugs. A family history of renal disease can suggest a hereditary disorder, especially polycystic kidney disease. Symptoms of itching, muscle cramps, anorexia, nausea, and even confusion are consistent with chronic renal impairment. Hemoptysis suggests a vasculitic disease, particularly antiglomerular basement membrane disease (Goodpasture's).

Examination

Carry out a full examination including blood pressure measurement, fundoscopy, examination for edema, and rectal and vaginal examinations where appropriate. Check for a distended bladder. Look for signs of systemic disease in all systems, especially neurological and rheumatological signs. Cardiac valve lesions raise the possibility of glomerulonephritis associated with infective endocarditis. Peripheral bruits or absent peripheral pulses indicate vascular disease and such patients are at risk of renal artery stenosis, which may result in renal artery bruits.

Kidneys

Enlarged kidneys may be palpable. The right kidney, which lies lower than the left because of the liver, is sometimes palpable when normal. To palpate the kidneys, place the right hand over the upper abdomen on the relevant side. On the same side, place the left hand with the fingers in the renal angle formed by the lateral margin of the lumbar muscles and the twelfth rib. As the patient inspires, push the fingers of the left hand anteriorly several times. You will feel an enlarged kidney with the right hand as it moves down the abdominal cavity during inspiration and is pushed anteriorly by the fingers of your left hand.

Fluid status

It is important to determine whether the patient has an excess or a deficiency of body water. Useful physical signs to look for include peripheral pitting edema, detectable especially at the ankles and sacrum, signs of pulmonary edema, effusions, the jugular venous pressure (JVP), and skin turgor. A cardiac gallop rhythm may suggest hypervolemia. A low blood pressure, especially with a postural drop (orthostatic hypertension), indicates hypovolemia.

Bedside investigation of urine

Dipstick test urine for hematuria, proteinuria, and glucosuria. If possible, use a microscope, ideally with phase contrast, to examine fresh urine. To concentrate cells or casts, centrifuge the urine and discard most of the supernatant.

Red cells. These can arise from anywhere in the urinary tract, but deformed (dysmorphic) red cells indicate glomerular bleeding.

White cells. These suggest inflammation, resulting from bacterial infection if they are polymorphonuclear cells or interstitial nephritis if they are eosinophils or lymphocytes.

Casts. These are cylindrical aggregates formed in the distal tubule or collecting ducts. *Red cell casts* indicate glomerular bleeding, usually due to glomerulonephritis. *White cell casts* suggest acute infection, usually bacterial. *Hyaline casts* and fine *granular casts* are normal findings. Hyaline casts are mainly protein and may be increased in proteinuria. Granular casts are also mainly protein. *Fatty casts* can occur in the nephrotic syndrome. *Waxy casts* are large and occur in dilated tubules in chronic renal failure.

Crystals. These may indicate a stone-forming tendency, but are not always of pathological significance because they can form after urine collection. Ideally, examine urine for crystals when it is fresh and at 37°C.

Infectious agents. Nitrites and leukocyte esterases on dipstick analysis suggest infection. Take a midstream urine sample for microscopy and culture.

Proteinuria. Quantify proteinuria. A spot albumin:creatinine ratio is the preferred investigation as it is more reliable than a total protein: creatinine ratio. At high levels of proteinuria, a spot urine protein:creatinine ratio or a 24-h urine collection can also be used.

5 The kidney: laboratory investigations and diagnostic imaging

Relationship between serum creatinine and renal function

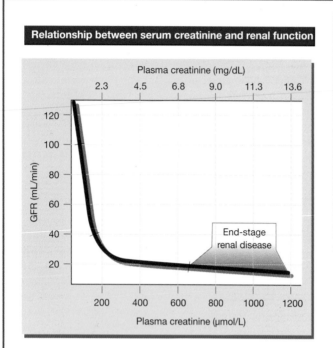

Estimating GFR

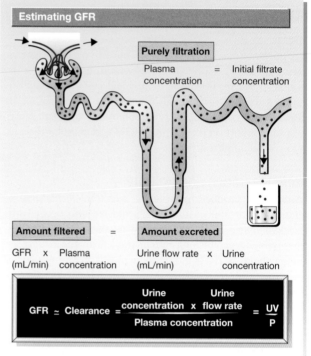

Purely filtration

| Plasma concentration | = | Initial filtrate concentration |

Amount filtered = **Amount excreted**

GFR × Plasma   Urine flow rate × Urine
(mL/min) concentration   (mL/min)   concentration

$$\text{GFR} \simeq \text{Clearance} = \frac{\text{Urine concentration} \times \text{Urine flow rate}}{\text{Plasma concentration}} = \frac{UV}{P}$$

Normal renal ultrasound scan

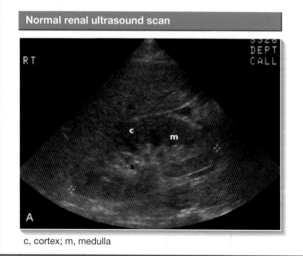

c, cortex; m, medulla

Cystic renal ultrasound scan

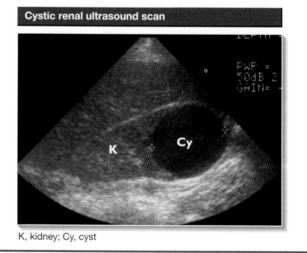

K, kidney; Cy, cyst

Blood tests

Take venous blood for routine biochemistry and hematology. A priority is to check that the serum potassium level is not dangerously elevated (see Chapter 18).

Estimating the glomerular filtration rate

Serum urea and creatinine

As urea and creatinine are excreted by the kidneys, they accumulate in the blood when renal function is impaired. However, because there is excess renal capacity, neither substance rises substantially until the glomerular filtration rate (GFR) falls to around 30 mL/min from a normal value of around 120 mL/min. **Urea** levels rise with a high protein intake or a catabolic state and fall with liver disease or overhydration. Urea is freely filtered, but there is also some tubular reabsorption, which is increased (along with sodium reabsorption) by dehydration or reduced renal perfusion, causing a greater elevation of urea than of creatinine. **Creatinine** is freely filtered, but there is also some tubular secretion. Creatinine is produced in muscle, and people with large muscle bulk can have higher values. Plasma **cystatin C** levels are more expensive to measure, but can provide better estimates of renal function than creatinine.

Clearance methods

When a substance is filtered, the initial concentration in the filtrate is the same as that in the plasma. If there is neither reabsorption nor secretion, then the quantity of the substance excreted in the final urine, in 1 min, is equal to the quantity removed from the plasma by filtration in 1 min. The amount excreted is calculated by multiplying the urine concentration by the urine flow rate per minute. This value must equal the plasma concentration multiplied by the GFR (volume of filtrate formed in 1 min). By measuring the plasma and urine concentration of a substance and the urine flow rate per minute, the GFR can be estimated.

Creatinine clearance provides a simple estimate of the GFR. A 24-h urine collection indicates urine flow rate in milliliters per minute. Creatinine clearance slightly overestimates the GFR because of tubular creatinine secretion. This secretion, and consequently the error, increase when the GFR is low. Cimetidine and trimethoprim inhibit creatinine secretion and so raise blood creatinine levels and reduce measured creatinine clearance. Inulin is neither secreted nor reabsorbed and is used to determine GFR accurately for research purposes. Algorithms such as the Chronic Kidney Disease Epidemiology Collaboration (CKD-EPI), modification of diet in renal disease (MDRD), and Cockcroft–Gault algorithms can predict creatinine clearance with useful accuracy from plasma creatinine and variables such as the patient's age, weight, and gender. These estimated GFRs (eGFRs) are discussed in Chapter 43.

Radio-isotope methods

GFR can be measured by following the fall in blood concentration of an injected substance such as ^{51}Cr-EDTA (chromium-51-labeled ethylenediaminetetra-acetic acid) or ^{99m}Tc-DTPA (technetium-99m-labeled diethylenetriaminepenta-acetic acid). These substances are removed only by the kidney. The rate of removal is estimated from serial plasma measurements and reflects the GFR.

Other biochemical investigations

Serum albumin levels are low in the nephrotic syndrome as a result of urinary protein loss. The nephrotic syndrome also causes hyperlipidemia. Electrophoresis of plasma proteins can demonstrate excess monoclonal immunoglobulins consistent with myeloma and other B-cell disorders. Urine electrophoresis may show leakage of free immunoglobulin light chains into the urine. Myoglobin in the blood or urine suggests rhabdomyolysis and free hemoglobin in the blood or urine suggests hemolysis. Free myoglobin and hemoglobin are both toxic to renal tubules. Arterial blood gases will reveal any acid-base disturbances.

Immunological investigations

A range of immunological and microbiological tests can be useful (see Chapters 32 and 42). Antineutrophil cytoplasmic antibodies (ANCA) suggest vasculitis and antiglomerular basement membrane antibodies suggest Goodpasture's syndrome. Antinuclear antibodies, antibodies to double-stranded DNA, and low complement levels suggest systemic lupus erythematosus.

Renal imaging

Ultrasonography provides information about renal size and anatomy, including the presence of cysts or calyceal dilation, suggesting obstruction. Doppler studies can be used to assess flow in the renal arteries and veins. Computed tomography (CT) and magnetic resonance imaging (MRI) can also visualize the renal system.

Plain radiography may reveal the renal size and detect radio-opaque stones. Intravenous contrast will produce an intravenous urogram (IVU), showing the renal outlines and the urinary tract. Unfortunately, the contrast can occasionally be nephrotoxic, particularly in dehydrated patients. Spiral CT scanning with intravenous contrast can produce excellent images of the entire renal tract, which are sometimes referred to as CT urograms.

The urinary tract can also be studied by injecting contrast up the ureters via the urethra and bladder or down the ureters by percutaneous puncture of the renal pelvis. Renal angiography can be performed using an arterial catheter inserted via the brachial or femoral artery to inject radio-opaque contrast into the renal arteries to visualize them.

Nuclear imaging

Scans using ^{99m}Tc-DTPA provide dynamic information about renal blood flow; scans with DMSA (dimercaptosuccinic acid) provide static information about localized renal function.

^{99m}Tc-DTPA is rapidly excreted by renal filtration and, after an intravenous bolus injection, the rise and fall of radioactivity over the kidney are detected and quantified with a gamma camera. The kinetics of these changes provide a good index of renal blood flow (see Chapter 8).

^{99m}Tc-DMSA localizes to proximal tubular cells, which take up succinate after intravenous injection; gamma camera images show the localization, shape, and function of each kidney separately.

Renal biopsy

Any histological diagnosis of renal disease requires renal biopsy. Percutaneous biopsy is performed with a long cutting needle through the back, usually with ultrasonic guidance. The major complication is bleeding. Rarely, an open biopsy is performed. The tissue obtained is examined by light microscopy, immunostaining using antibodies to complement or immunoglobulins, and often electron microscopy.

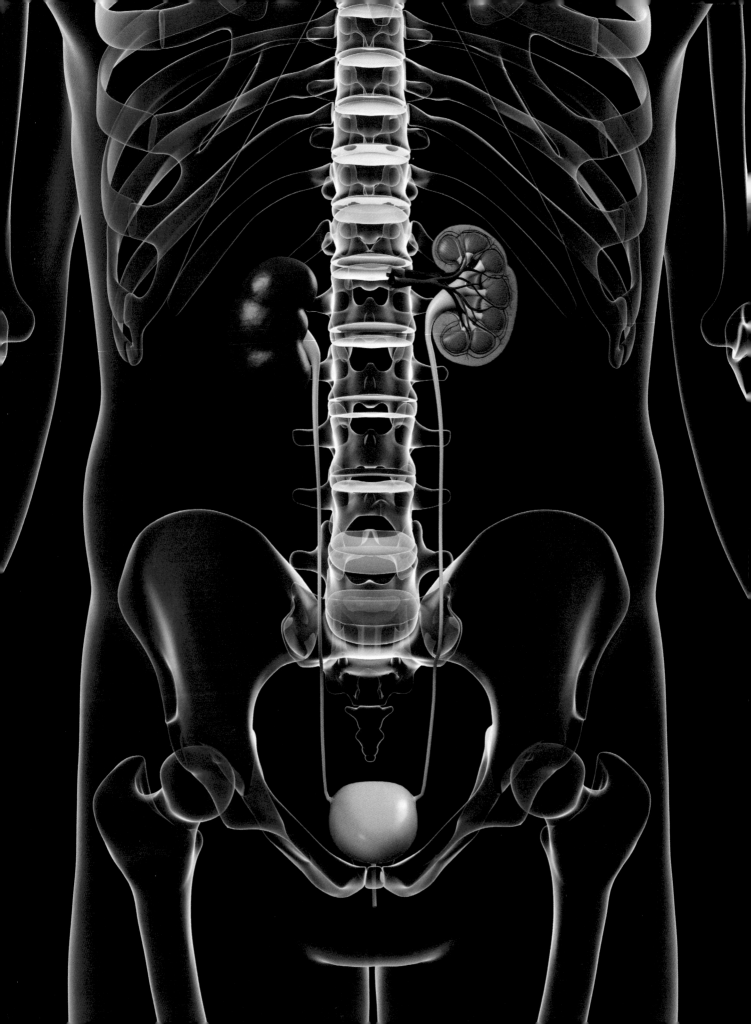

Filtration and blood flow

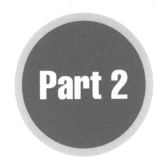

Part 2

Chapters

6 **Renal vascular biology** 14
7 **Glomerular filtration** 16
8 **Renal vascular disease** 18
9 **Erythropoietin and anemia in renal disease** 20

 Don't forget to visit the companion website for this book
www.ataglanceseries.com/renalsystem

6 Renal vascular biology

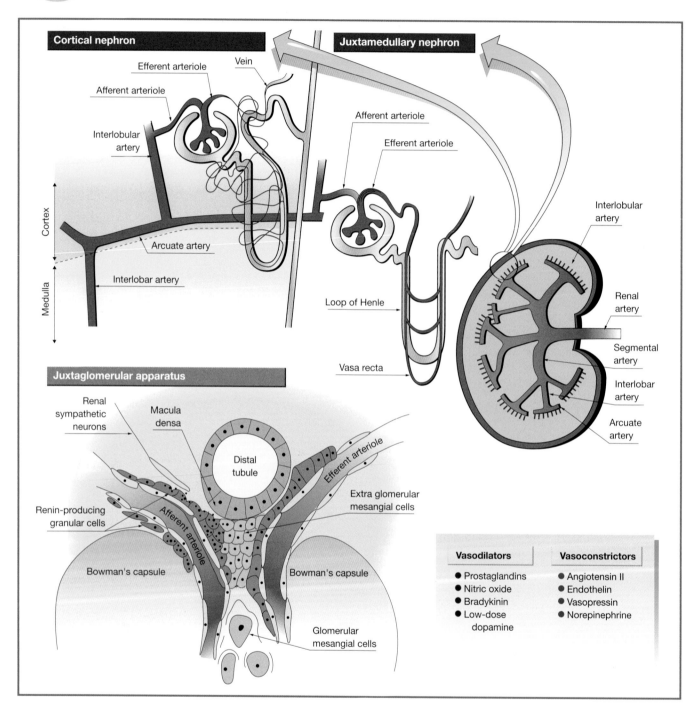

Cortical nephron

Efferent arteriole
Vein
Afferent arteriole
Interlobular artery
Cortex
Arcuate artery
Medulla
Interlobar artery

Juxtamedullary nephron

Afferent arteriole
Efferent arteriole
Loop of Henle
Vasa recta

Interlobular artery
Renal artery
Segmental artery
Interlobar artery
Arcuate artery

Juxtaglomerular apparatus

Renal sympathetic neurons
Macula densa
Distal tubule
Efferent arteriole
Extra glomerular mesangial cells
Renin-producing granular cells
Afferent arteriole
Bowman's capsule
Bowman's capsule
Glomerular mesangial cells

Vasodilators	Vasoconstrictors
● Prostaglandins	● Angiotensin II
● Nitric oxide	● Endothelin
● Bradykinin	● Vasopressin
● Low-dose dopamine	● Norepinephrine

The Renal System at a Glance, Fourth Edition. Chris O'Callaghan. © 2017 John Wiley & Sons, Ltd. Published 2017 by John Wiley & Sons, Ltd.
Companion website: www.ataglanceseries.com/renalsystem

Each kidney is supplied by a renal artery arising from the aorta. Within the kidney, the renal artery divides into two or three segmental arteries, which further subdivide into interlobar arteries and then into arcuate arteries. The arcuate arteries curve parallel to the outer surface of the kidney, giving rise to the interlobular arteries, which ascend through the cortex and give off the afferent arterioles that supply the glomerular capillary bed. Beyond the glomeruli, the capillaries regroup as efferent arterioles. In the outer cortex, these give rise to peritubular capillaries which surround the tubules. Efferent arterioles arising from the juxtamedullary nephrons descend into the medulla and give rise to the vasa recta, which descend and re-ascend in close proximity to the loops of Henle. Blood leaves the kidney in veins that travel with the corresponding arteries and join to form a single renal vein, which enters the inferior vena cava.

Renal blood flow

Together the kidneys receive a renal blood flow (**RBF**) of 1000 mL/min, which is 20% of the cardiac output. The normal hematocrit is 0.45, so red cells account for 45% of RBF, and the renal plasma flow (**RPF**) is 550 mL/min. The glomerular filtration rate (**GFR**) is about 120 mL/min, so the filtration fraction (**FF** = GFR/RPF), which is the proportion of plasma that is filtered, is around 20%. Renal vascular resistance arises mainly from the afferent and efferent arterioles. High pressure in the glomerular capillaries forces filtrate through the filtration barrier. This pressure is reduced by afferent arteriolar constriction and increased by efferent arteriolar constriction.

Measuring renal blood and plasma flow

The amount of a substance removed from plasma by the kidneys in 1 min (arterial–venous concentration × RPF) equals the amount appearing in the urine in 1 min (urine flow/min × urine concentration). If arterial, venous, and urinary concentration and urine flow are measured, RPF can be calculated. This can be done after an injection of *p*-aminohippuric acid (PAH), which is fully removed after a single pass through the kidney. RBF can be calculated from the RPF if the hematocrit is known:

$$RBF = RPF/(1 - Hematocrit)$$

99mTc-labeled DTPA (diethylenetriaminepenta-acetic acid) and MAG$_3$ (mercaptoacetyltriglycine) are both removed by the kidney so, in clinical practice, they can be detected by a gamma camera to estimate RBF.

Regulation of renal blood flow

Autoregulation

- *Myogenic reflex.* A rise in pressure stretches the blood vessel, causing reflex vasoconstriction, which reduces flow.
- *Tubuloglomerular feedback.* A rise in glomerular pressure increases GFR and, therefore, tubular flow rate. This reduces the time available for sodium and chloride reabsorption in the ascending loop of Henle.

The higher tubular sodium and chloride concentrations detected by the macula densa cause the juxtaglomerular apparatus (JGA) to release **adenosine**. Adenosine acts predominantly on A1 receptors to cause afferent arteriolar vasoconstriction, which reduces GFR. Adenosine also promotes proximal tubule sodium reabsorption.

Renin–angiotensin II system

The JGA releases renin in response to a drop in afferent arteriolar pressure, a fall in tubular flow rate, or a fall in tubular sodium and chloride concentration at the macula densa. Other stimuli include sympathetic nerve stimulation of β$_1$-adrenergic receptors on granular cells and a fall in angiotensin II (AngII) levels. **Renin** promotes production of **AngII** which acts via AT1 (type 1 angiotensin II receptors) to vasoconstrict afferent and efferent arterioles. The dominant effect is on efferent arteriolar constriction, so the GFR is increased.

Prostaglandins

Many peripheral vasoconstrictors, especially AngII, vasopressin, endothelin, and norepinephrine (noradrenaline) stimulate the renal production of vasodilating prostaglandins such as PGE2 and PGI2 (prostacyclin). This protects the kidney from severe vasoconstriction.

Vasoactive peptides

- *Bradykinin* is a peptide of nine amino acids released from a precursor kallidin by the enzyme kallikrein in the distal tubule and glomerulus. It acts on B$_1$- and B$_2$-receptors, promoting prostaglandin synthesis and vasodilation.
- *Natriuretic peptides* (ANP, BNP, and CNP) are released from cardiac cells and can produce systemic vasodilation via natriuretic peptide receptors (NPRs).
- *Endothelin* is a peptide of 21 amino acids made in renal vascular endothelial cells and tubules. It is a potent vasoconstrictor. It acts via the phosphoinositide messenger system and promotes calcium entry into cells. In the periphery, endothelin acts mainly on ET$_A$-receptors; in the kidney, it acts mainly on ET$_B$-receptors.
- *Vasopressin (ADH)* promotes vasoconstriction via V$_1$-receptors and antidiuretic action via V$_2$-receptors.
- *Adrenomedullin* promotes renal vasodilation and is produced in the kidney.

Other regulatory pathways

- *Renal nerves* contain sympathetic neurons which release norepinephrine (noradrenaline). Like circulating epinephrine (adrenaline), this acts via G-protein-linked α$_1$-receptors, causing constriction of afferent and efferent arterioles. Renin release is also promoted.
- *Dopamine* is sometimes used clinically to promote RBF. At low concentrations (1–3 μg/kg/min), it has a vasodilatory effect through DA$_1$-receptors acting via cAMP. At higher concentrations, dopamine causes renal vasoconstriction via α$_1$-receptors and through β$_1$-receptor-mediated renin release.
- *Nitric oxide (NO)* is a potent vasodilator that acts via cGMP and regulates renal vascular smooth muscle tone. It is synthesized from L-arginine by NO synthases in the macula densa, endothelium, and mesangial cells. It has a short half-life and is upregulated in response to mechanical sheer stress.
- *Adenosine* produces vasoconstriction via A$_1$-receptors and vasodilation via A$_2$-receptors.

7 Glomerular filtration

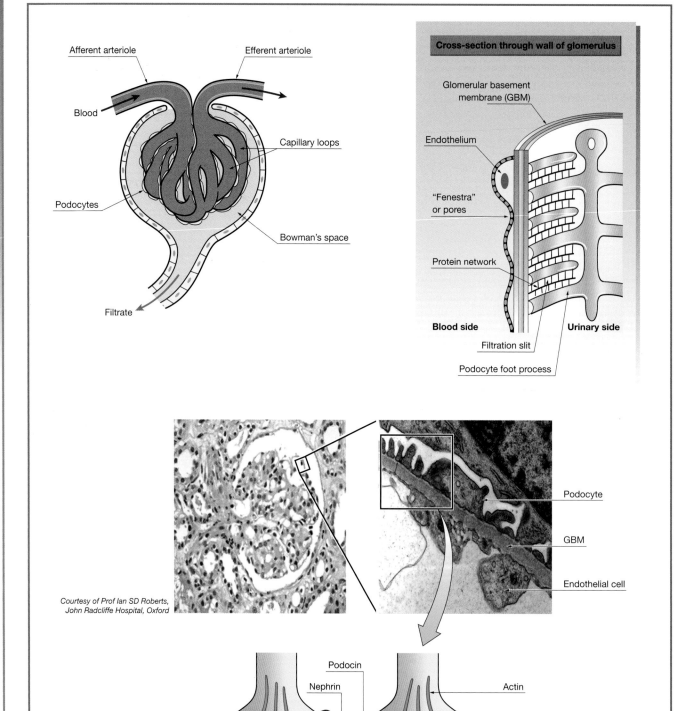

Cross-section through wall of glomerulus

Afferent arteriole

Efferent arteriole

Blood

Capillary loops

Podocytes

Bowman's space

Filtrate

Glomerular basement membrane (GBM)

Endothelium

"Fenestra" or pores

Protein network

Blood side

Filtration slit

Podocyte foot process

Urinary side

Courtesy of Prof Ian SD Roberts, John Radcliffe Hospital, Oxford

Podocyte

GBM

Endothelial cell

Podocin

Nephrin

Actin

Foot process

Integrins

GBM

Fenestrated endothelial cell

The Renal System at a Glance, Fourth Edition. Chris O'Callaghan. © 2017 John Wiley & Sons, Ltd. Published 2017 by John Wiley & Sons, Ltd.
Companion website: www.ataglanceseries.com/renalsystem

Blood entering the renal arteries is eventually channeled through an afferent arteriole to the glomerular capillary bed. This highly specialized capillary network forms a ball-like structure or glomerulus in which filtration occurs. The glomerular capillary endothelial cells are relatively flat cells with the capillary lumen on one side and a specialized basement membrane on the other side of the cells known as the glomerular basement membrane. Unlike normal capillaries elsewhere in the body, the glomerular capillaries are not surrounded by interstitial fluid. Instead, on the opposite side of the basement membrane are epithelial cells that form the inner surface of Bowman's capsule. These tubular epithelial cells are known as podocytes because of their "foot processes" and are highly specialized. During embryonic development, each glomerular capillary invaginates a developing tubule to form a glomerulus. Consequently, each mature glomerular capillary is surrounded by the tubular collecting system. Filtration occurs within the glomerulus and the filtered fluid passes from the glomerular capillary lumen into the tubular system. The space immediately beyond the filtration barrier into which the filtered fluid passes is known as Bowman's space. The glomerulus also contains mesangial cells which have both contractile and phagocytic properties and appear to serve a structural role in supporting the capillary loops. Approaches for measuring and estimating GFR are discussed in Chapters 5 and 43.

The filtration barrier

The filtration barrier consists of three components, the glomerular endothelial cells, the glomerular basement membrane, and the podocytes. The glomerular endothelial cells are thin and have pores within them of around 70–100 nm which are filled with negatively charged proteins, predominantly podocalyxin. The glomerular basement membrane is a complex network of glycoproteins. The three-dimensional scaffold of this complex is composed of helical strands of type 4 collagen on which the other components are attached. These other proteins include heparan sulfate proteoglycan, laminin, podocalyxin, fibronectin, and entactin.

The glomerular basement membrane has three layers known, from the endothelial side to the epithelial side, as the lamina densa, lamina rara interna, and lamina rara externa. The lamina densa is a dense and relatively homogeneous layer, but the two lamina rara layers are less dense and have a significant negative charge. In Alport's syndrome (Chapter 34) collagen mutations affect the glomerular basement membrane structure and cause kidney disease.

The epithelial cells or podocytes lining Bowman's space are highly specialized with well-developed foot processes which are attached to the tubular side of the glomerular basement membrane. Foot processes from different podocytes interdigitate, but do not touch each other. Between the interdigitating foot processes are spaces known as a filtration slits which are around 25–65 nm across. A network of proteins associated with the podocytes foot processes forms "slit pores" across these slits. The major protein in the slit pores is nephrin and this is associated with other proteins including NEPH1, P-cadherin, CD2AP, ZO-1, and podocin. Podocin plays a role in regulating the movement of the transmembrane protein nephrin to the slit pores. Integrins help to attach the podocytes to the glomerular basement membrane. Mutations in the podocyte proteins nephrin or podocin can cause congenital nephrotic syndrome. Focal segmental glomerulosclerosis with proteinuria can arise from mutations in alpha-actinin-4 and INF2 which lead to podocyte dysfunction through their effects on the podocyte actin cytoskeleton.

The filtration process

Filtration takes place because the hydraulic pressure gradient between the glomerular capillaries and Bowman's space exceeds the opposing oncotic pressure gradient. The hydraulic pressure in the glomerulus is influenced by the state of vasoconstriction of both the afferent and efferent arterioles. The oncotic pressure gradient reflects the difference in the concentration of osmotically active components between plasma and the filtered fluid in Bowman's capsule. As larger plasma proteins are not filtered in the glomerulus, the oncotic pressure gradient tends to oppose filtration.

The multiple layers of the filtration barrier provide a matrix through which size and charge selection occurs during glomerular filtration, but there is debate about the precise role of each layer of the barrier. The high pressure in the glomerulus forces water and solutes through the molecular sieve formed by the filtration barrier. The extent of their filtration depends to some extent upon their electrical charge and to a larger extent upon size. Neutral particles above 4.2 nm are not filtered, but negatively charged particles are more restricted and are not filtered if they are over 3.4 nm. Both size and charge selectivity can be lost in disease states, especially the nephrotic syndrome (Chapter 35).

Regulation of filtration

Afferent arteriolar constriction reduces glomerular capillary pressure and so lowers glomerular filtration. Efferent arteriolar constriction raises glomerular capillary pressure and so increases glomerular filtration. There is substantial renal autoregulation, such that if systemic blood pressure falls and renal perfusion pressure fall, GFR is maintained by efferent arteriolar constriction. The mechanisms involved include a myogenic reflex in which vascular smooth muscle respond to stretch and tubuloglomerular feedback involving the macula densa (Chapter 6). In addition, multiple factors also influence filtration through effects on renal arteriolar tone (Chapter 40).

8 Renal vascular disease

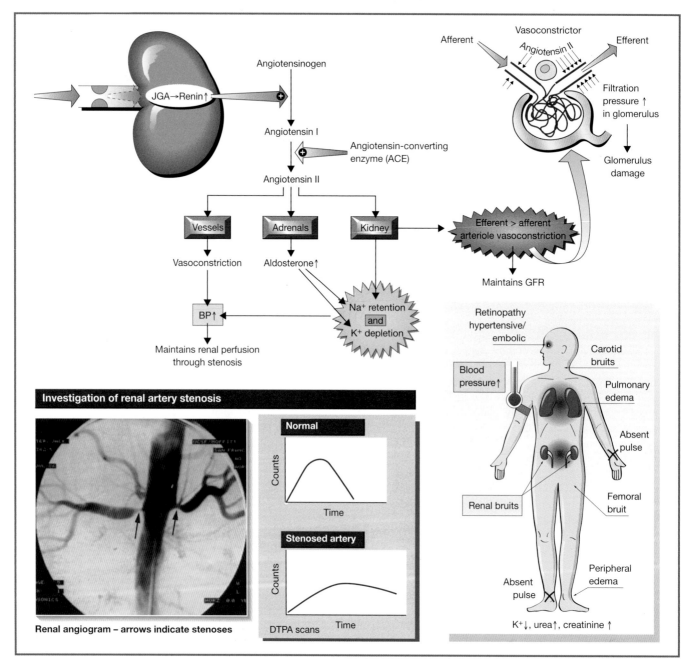

Investigation of renal artery stenosis

Renal angiogram – arrows indicate stenoses

Normal

Counts

Time

Stenosed artery

Counts

Time

DTPA scans

Retinopathy hypertensive/embolic

Blood pressure↑

Carotid bruits

Pulmonary edema

Absent pulse

Renal bruits

Femoral bruit

Absent pulse

Peripheral edema

K+↓, urea↑, creatinine ↑

Renal artery stenosis reduces the renal blood flow and glomerular filtration, causing renal ischemia, hypertension, and sodium and water retention. The main causes are atherosclerosis in older patients and fibromuscular dysplasia in young patients. Renal artery stenosis accounts for 1–5% of all hypertension. Atherosclerotic disease is often bilateral and usually progresses, sometimes to complete occlusion. Fibromuscular dysplasia does not usually cause occlusion.

Renal artery stenosis

Pathophysiology

Hypertension

Decreased renal perfusion stimulates the juxtaglomerular apparatus to release renin, which enhances angiotensin II production. Angiotensin II causes hypertension by systemic

The Renal System at a Glance, Fourth Edition. Chris O'Callaghan. © 2017 John Wiley & Sons, Ltd. Published 2017 by John Wiley & Sons, Ltd.
Companion website: www.ataglanceseries.com/renalsystem

vasoconstriction and by stimulating aldosterone release, which promotes salt and water retention.

Renal impairment

Angiotensin II vasoconstricts the efferent arterioles more than the afferent arterioles. This reduces renal blood flow, but maintains glomerular filtration, so the filtration fraction is increased. Inhibition of angiotensin II (with angiotensin-converting enzyme inhibitors or angiotensin II receptor blockers) removes the efferent arteriolar constriction, causing a fall in the glomerular filtration rate (GFR). Microembolization from an atheromatous plaque can contribute to renal damage. If only one kidney has a stenosed artery, plasma creatinine may be normal because of compensatory hyperfiltration by the other kidney.

Edema

Bilateral renal artery disease causes enhanced proximal tubular sodium reabsorption. Contributory factors include a fall in renal blood flow, stimulation of the proximal tubule NHE3 Na^+/H^+ exchanger by angiotensin II, and stimulation of distal tubular sodium reabsorption by aldosterone. Aldosterone also promotes potassium secretion, which can cause hypokalemia unless there is renal impairment. Mild proteinuria can occur, possibly because angiotensin II increases glomerular pore size. In unilateral renal artery stenosis, salt and water balance are normalized by the other kidney.

Etiology of renal artery stenosis

Atherosclerotic disease usually affects the proximal renal artery and accounts for most cases. There is often vascular disease elsewhere and the usual risk factors for atherosclerosis—smoking, diabetes mellitus, hypertension, a family history, and hyperlipidemia. **Fibromuscular dysplasia** occurs in younger patients, especially women. It can occur as multiple bands separated by dilated segments, appearing like a string of beads on an angiogram. **Rare causes** of renal artery stenosis include the large vessel vasculitis Takayasu arteritis (TAK), neurofibromatosis, pressure from renal artery aneurysms, and extrinsic pressure.

History and examination

There may be a history of risk factors for atherosclerosis or symptoms of vascular disease elsewhere. A rapid deterioration in renal function caused by an ACE inhibitor (ACEI) or angiotensin receptor blocker is highly suggestive. There are often hypertension and signs of vascular disease elsewhere, such as absent pulses, aneurysms, or arterial bruits. Bruits, caused by turbulent flow through a stenosed renal artery, may be heard over the kidneys. There may be hypertensive retinopathy and pulmonary or peripheral edema.

Investigation

The diagnosis is suggested by hypokalemia, elevated urea and creatinine, and different-sized kidneys on ultrasonography. With unilateral disease, ischemic damage reduces the size of the affected kidney. The definitive investigation is angiography through an arterial catheter introduced at the groin or in the arm. Noninvasive imaging techniques such as magnetic resonance angiography and Doppler ultrasonography are improving, and magnetic resonance angiography is commonly used to identify renal artery stenosis. ^{99m}**Tc-labeled DTPA** (technetium-99m-labeled diethylenetriaminepenta-acetic acid) is freely filtered at the glomerulus and neither secreted nor reabsorbed. After injection, a gamma camera produces a curve showing isotope accumulation in each kidney. In renal artery stenosis, angiotensin II increases proximal tubular sodium and therefore water reabsorption (see Chapter 10). This reduces urine flow, which delays the peak and slows the downward phase. Furosemide given during the scan increases the specificity for enhanced proximal reabsorption by inhibiting excess distal salt reabsorption. Administration of an ACE inhibitor during the renogram removes the effect of angiotensin II (which also maintains the GFR) and makes the test more sensitive.

Treatment

ACE inhibitors and angiotensin receptor blockers can reduce the GFR, and a unilateral fall in GFR may be undetected by serum creatinine measurement. They can help blood pressure control, but require careful monitoring. Aspirin may prevent thrombus formation at the stenosis and statin drugs can reduce the progression of atherosclerotic lesions. Percutaneous transluminal balloon angioplasty, sometimes with the insertion of an expandable stent, can be undertaken, but trial results do not indicate substantial benefit. The response of hypertension to relief of the stenosis is variable, and it usually does not have a beneficial impact on renal function. With atherosclerotic disease, balloon angioplasty can dislodge atherosclerotic material that may deposit in the kidney, impairing kidney function. Very rarely, uncontrollable hypertension requires renal embolization or nephrectomy to remove the source of renin. The success rate is higher for fibromuscular dysplasia, is better than for atherosclerotic disease, and balloon angioplasty is usually undertaken in this situation.

Cholesterol emboli

Detached fragments of atheroma in the aorta or renal arteries can embolize to the kidneys, especially after arterial surgery or angiographic instrumentation. Microemboli of cholesterol crystals and debris can provoke inflammation and fibrosis. Showers of these crystals can also cause *livedo reticularis* in the legs or microembolic lesions in the retina.

Renal vein thrombosis

Thrombus in the renal veins or their tributaries reduces the renal blood flow and impairs renal function. This may be clinically silent, although flank pain, loin tenderness, and macroscopic hematuria can occur. Diagnosis is made by renal venography, but may be evident using Doppler flow studies or computed tomography or magnetic resonance imaging. Any prothrombotic state can cause renal vein thrombosis. In nephrotic syndrome, renal vein thrombosis impairs renal function, increases proteinuria, and almost always causes microscopic hematuria. Renal vein thrombosis can extend and occlude the inferior vena cava or cause pulmonary emboli.

Erythropoietin and anemia in renal disease

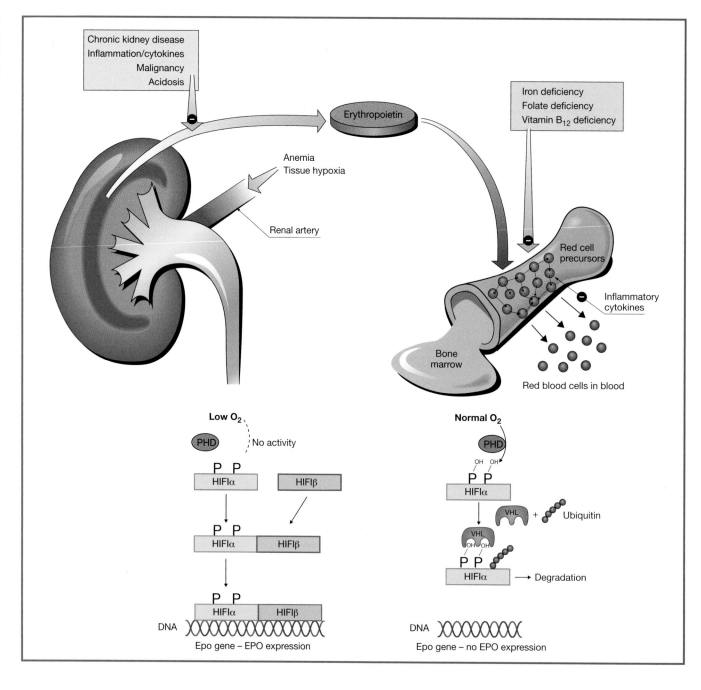

The kidney is the main source of erythropoietin, the hematopoietic growth factor that promotes red blood cell formation. Erythropoietin increases reticulocyte production and early release of reticulocytes from the bone marrow. In chronic renal failure, erythropoietin production is inadequate and there is usually anemia.

Mature erythropoietin (**EPO**) is a heavily glycosylated protein consisting of 165 amino acids. It interacts with the erythropoietin receptor (**EpoR**), which is homologous to other growth factor receptors. Binding of erythropoietin to its receptor results in receptor internalization, and subsequent signaling events include tyrosine phosphorylation and calcium entry. The receptor is expressed on early erythroid progenitor cells and the level of expression increases during red cell development. Withdrawal of erythropoietin from these precursor cells causes apoptotic cell death.

The Renal System at a Glance, Fourth Edition. Chris O'Callaghan. © 2017 John Wiley & Sons, Ltd. Published 2017 by John Wiley & Sons, Ltd.
Companion website: www.ataglanceseries.com/renalsystem

Erythropoietin production

The major site of erythropoietin production in the adult is the kidney. A small amount is also produced by the liver in some hepatocytes and in fibroblastoid Ito cells; the liver is the major site of production in the fetus and neonate. In the kidney, erythropoietin is made in type I fibroblastoid cells in the peritubular interstitium of the cortex and outer medulla. There is normally a low basal level of erythropoietin production by the kidney, but this is enhanced by anemia or a fall in arterial PO_2, situations that both cause tissue hypoxia. Hypoxia initially stimulates erythropoietin mRNA synthesis in cells in the deep cortex, but as hypoxia progresses, cells in more superficial sites also produce erythropoietin. This distribution reflects advancing hypoxia as there is a gradient of hypoxia from the cortex to the inner medulla because the medulla receives all its blood supply from the vasa recta.

Low erythropoietin levels in response to anemia are found in chronic renal failure, inflammatory disease, malignancy, acidosis, and starvation, or with the use of angiotensin-converting enzyme inhibitors. Acidosis reduces the oxygen affinity of hemoglobin, which can promote tissue oxygenation and so reduce the stimulus to erythropoietin production. In inflammatory disease, cytokines such as tumor necrosis factor-α reduce erythropoietin production, and cytokines such as interferon-β suppress the erythropoietic response to erythropoietin.

Hypoxic stimulation of erythropoietin production

When oxygen levels are low, the transcription factor protein **HIF1** (hypoxia inducible factor 1) binds to the erythropoietin gene to promote its expression. HIF1 consists of two components, HIF1α and HIF1β. However, when oxygen levels are normal, oxygen-dependent prolyl hydroxylase domain enzymes (PHDs) add hydroxyl groups to proline residues in the HIF1α protein. These hydroxyprolines are recognized by the **VHL** (von Hippel–Lindau) protein which, in complex with other proteins, can then attach ubiquitin groups to HIF1α, triggering its destruction by the proteasome. Thus, when oxygen levels are normal, HIF1α is rapidly degraded, but when oxygen levels are low, proline hydroxylation does not occur and HIF1α is stable and can combine with HIF1β to activate the erythropoietin gene. In addition, normal oxygen levels also promote hydroxylation of asparagine residues in HIF1α by the FIH1 enzyme and this impairs HIF1α function. The PHD enzymes require iron to function efficiently.

Erythropoietin and chronic renal failure

Anemia is common in advanced chronic kidney disease, but most patients do not have a raised erythropoietin level. Chronic kidney disease often causes interstitial changes, and the type I erythropoietin-producing cells become more myofibroblastoid with less potential for erythropoietin production. Although there may be some destruction of these erythropoietin-producing cells, the main problem is a failure of the cells to produce enough erythropoietin in response to the anemia. An exception is polycystic kidney disease, where erythropoietin production is often preserved or even elevated and erythropoietin production has been demonstrated in cyst wall cells.

Other factors in chronic kidney disease, such as reduced red cell survival, can contribute to the anemia, which is characteristically normocytic/normochromic. However, it is always important to exclude iron deficiency resulting from poor intake or blood loss and to exclude folate deficiency or, less commonly, vitamin B_{12} deficiency. The serum ferritin level should be measured to exclude iron deficiency, but can be spuriously elevated if there is inflammation. Aluminum toxicity can cause a microcytic anemia like that of iron deficiency, and can be a problem in patients who have used aluminum-containing phosphate-binding agents.

Red cell production requires iron which can only exit cells in the gut or elsewhere via the ferroportin iron transporter. In chronic kidney disease factors including inflammation increase the production of hepcidin from the liver and this circulating hepcidin binds to ferroportin and blocks iron exit. This reduces gut iron absorption, lowers the iron supply for red cell production and contributes to anemia.

Erythropoietin therapy

Renal transplantation restores normal erythropoietin production, although continued erythropoietin production from the native kidneys can cause polycythemia. Generally, patients on peritoneal dialysis have less anemia than those on hemodialysis, but in both cases, erythropoietin is given to maintain a normal hemoglobin level.

Subcutaneous administration gives a more sustained rise in erythropoietin level than intravenous administration and is usually given one to three times weekly. Darbepoetin is a form of erythropoietin that has extra glycosylation and can be given just once weekly because the extra sugar content increases its half-life. Erythropoietin can cause hypertension or polycythemia, so the blood count and blood pressure are checked every 2 weeks. The dose is adjusted upward if there is no response by 4 weeks. A good response to therapy is first indicated by a rise in the reticulocyte count. When the target hemoglobin is reached, it may be possible to reduce the dose. It is important that sufficient iron is available during erythropoietin therapy—ferritin, transferrin saturation, and the appearance of hypochromic cells on the blood film are useful guides to iron levels. Intravenous iron therapy may be required.

The major complications are polycythemia, hypertension, and thrombosis of vascular access sites used for dialysis. Resistance to erythropoietin therapy often reflects iron deficiency, inflammation, or malignancy. Severe hyperparathyroidism can blunt the response to erythropoietin, possibly because of bone marrow fibrosis. New PHD enzyme inhibitors stabilize HIF1α, thus promoting erythropoietin expression, and show promise in the treatment of anemia in chronic kidney disease.

Acute renal failure

In acute renal failure, anemia usually represents blood loss or hemolysis. Although erythropoietin levels often fail to rise appropriately, the patients are usually unwell, often with ongoing sepsis or inflammation, which renders erythropoietin ineffective.

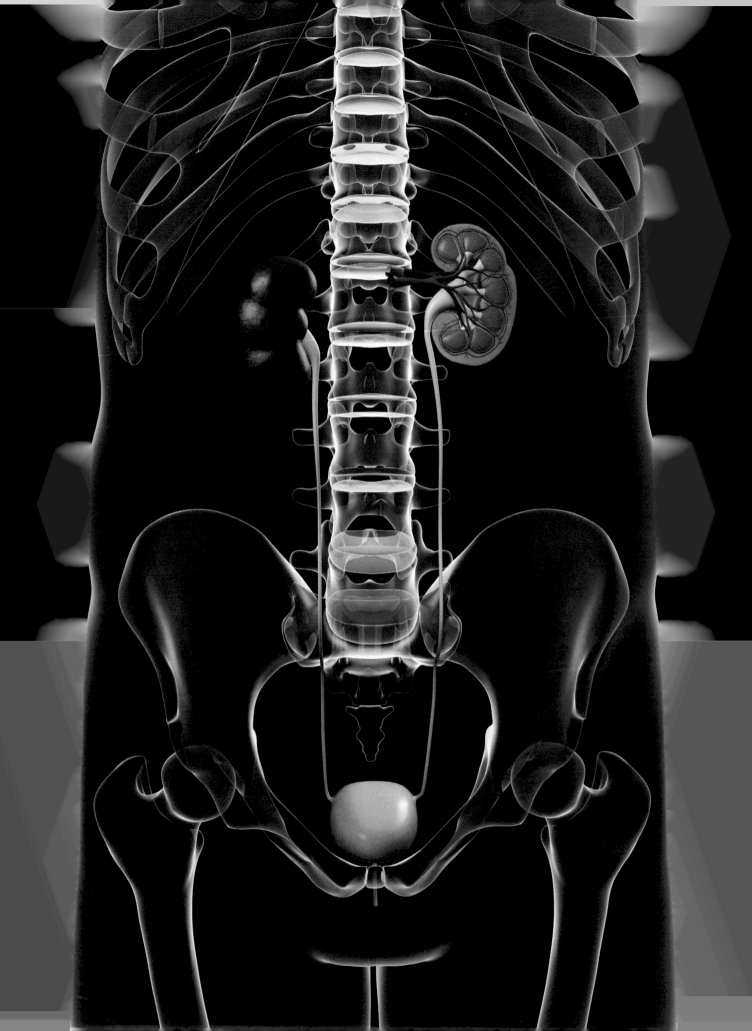

Sodium and water

Part 3

Chapters

10 Renal sodium handling 24
11 The kidney and water handling 26
12 Regulation of body sodium and body water 28
13 Disorders of sodium and water metabolism 30
14 Hyponatremia and hypernatremia 32
15 The edema states: sodium and water
    retention 34

 Don't forget to visit the companion website for this book
www.ataglanceseries.com/renalsystem

10 Renal sodium handling

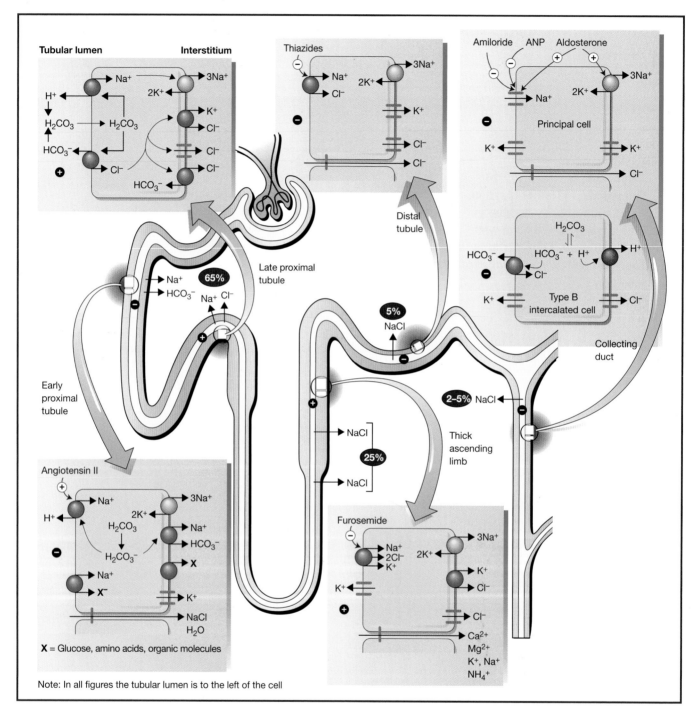

X = Glucose, amino acids, organic molecules

Note: In all figures the tubular lumen is to the left of the cell

The Renal System at a Glance, Fourth Edition. Chris O'Callaghan. © 2017 John Wiley & Sons, Ltd. Published 2017 by John Wiley & Sons, Ltd.
Companion website: www.ataglanceseries.com/renalsystem

Sodium is the major extracellular cation and its concentration is tightly controlled. Sodium and chloride ions are freely filtered in the glomerulus, so the concentration of these ions in the filtrate is similar to that in blood (135–145 mmol/L for sodium). Daily dietary sodium chloride intake is usually 2–10 g, but the daily filtrate volume of around 200 L contains about 2 kg of sodium chloride. The kidney therefore reabsorbs a huge amount of salt in the proximal tubules and the loop of Henle. The little that is left is reabsorbed in a precisely regulated manner by the distal tubules and collecting ducts, to maintain accurate salt balance. About 5% of the salt intake is lost in sweat and feces.

The basolateral membranes of the tubular cells contain Na^+/K^+ ATPases that actively pump sodium into the peritubular plasma. From here, sodium ions pass freely into the blood to complete the reabsorption process. The continual pumping of sodium out of the cells and its subsequent removal by the blood creates a Na^+ gradient between the tubular filtrate and the cell cytoplasm. This gradient allows Na^+ from the filtrate to enter the cells passively at their apical membrane, provided that suitable channels or transporters are present.

Sodium handling along the nephron

Proximal tubule

Of the filtered sodium, 65% is reabsorbed in the proximal tubule. In the early proximal tubule, a large amount of reabsorption takes place, but the cell junctions are slightly leaky, limiting the concentration gradient that can be established between the filtrate and the peritubular plasma. In the late proximal tubule, the transport rate is lower, but tight junctions allow a larger gradient to be established.

In the early tubule, the sodium gradient drives the co-transport of sodium with bicarbonate, amino acids, glucose, or other organic molecules. The Na^+/H^+ exchanger (**NHE3**) uses the sodium gradient to drive sodium reabsorption from the filtrate and H^+ secretion into the filtrate. As carbonic anhydrase is present in the cell cytoplasm and tubular lumen, the secretion of H^+ is equivalent to the reabsorption of bicarbonate (HCO_3^-) (see Chapters 19 and 20). The apical secretion of H^+ is balanced by the basolateral exit of bicarbonate with sodium. Chloride concentration rises along the proximal tubule. When the positively charged sodium ions leave the lumen with neutral organic molecules, the lumen is left with a negative charge. This repels negatively charged chloride ions, which leave the lumen through the paracellular route between the cells.

By the time the filtrate reaches the late proximal tubule, most organic molecules and bicarbonate have already been removed and sodium ions are reabsorbed mainly with chloride ions. The Na^+/H^+ exchanger works in parallel to a chloride/base anion exchanger (**AE1**) and, as the base—usually bicarbonate, formate, or oxalate—is recycled across the apical membrane, the overall effect is that sodium chloride is reabsorbed. Chloride ions leave the cell alone or in exchange for another negatively charged ion or in co-transport with potassium. The higher tubular chloride concentration promotes chloride-coupled reabsorption.

The loop of Henle

The thin and thick ascending portions of the loop of Henle together reabsorb 25% of the filtered sodium.

Thin segments

Cells in the walls of the thin segments of the loop are thin and flat epithelial cells. No active transport occurs here and there are few mitochondria. The thin descending segment is permeable to water but not to sodium, so water leaves the tubule passively to enter the hypertonic medullary interstitium. In contrast, the thin ascending limb is permeable to sodium but not to water. As the filtrate loses water in the descending limb, there is a high concentration of sodium and chloride ions in the lumen of the thin ascending limb, and both ions diffuse out.

Thick ascending limb

The cells of the thick segment of the loop are large, with multiple mitochondria that generate energy for the active transport of sodium ions.

The key transport molecule is the **NKCC2** transporter, which uses the sodium gradient for the co-transport of one sodium, one potassium, and two chloride ions. As the potassium ion can re-enter the tubule via an ROMK channel, the net effect is the removal of one sodium and two chloride ions, leaving the tubular lumen positively charged. This positive potential drives the paracellular transport of positively charged ions, including sodium, potassium, calcium, magnesium, and ammonium. The NKCC2 transporter has multiple transmembrane domains and is inhibited by the diuretic furosemide (see Chapter 29).

Distal tubule

The distal tubule reabsorbs a further 5% of the filtered sodium. This transport occurs via the **NCC**, sodium chloride co-transport protein that is inhibited by the thiazide diuretics. As the fluid in the lumen in this portion of the nephron is negative, there is also some paracellular movement of negatively charged chloride ions.

Collecting tubules and ducts

Around 2–5% of filtered sodium is reabsorbed in the collecting ducts, which contain two characteristic cell types.

• **The principal cells.** Sodium enters these cells via the epithelial sodium channel (**ENaC**), leaving the lumen negatively charged. This negative charge drives the paracellular movement of chloride. The ENaC is composed of three homologous subunits and is inhibited by the diuretic drug amiloride.

• **The type B intercalated cells.** These have no Na^+/K^+ ATPase but do have an H^+ ATPase, which establishes a hydrogen ion gradient. The energy required for the transport function of these cells is derived from this H^+ gradient instead of the usual Na^+ gradient. As H^+ ions are removed from the cell, the net result is the secretion of bicarbonate coupled to the reabsorption of chloride (see Chapter 20).

Sodium reabsorption by principal cells and chloride reabsorption by the intercalated cells are the final stages in sodium chloride reabsorption before urine leaves the kidney.

11 The kidney and water handling

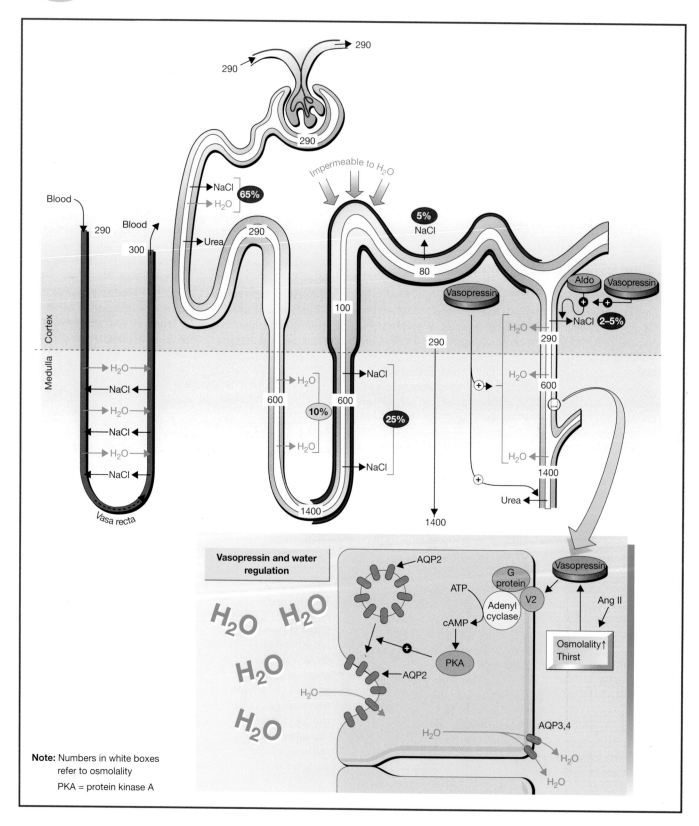

Note: Numbers in white boxes refer to osmolality

PKA = protein kinase A

The Renal System at a Glance, Fourth Edition. Chris O'Callaghan. © 2017 John Wiley & Sons, Ltd. Published 2017 by John Wiley & Sons, Ltd.

Companion website: www.ataglanceseries.com/renalsystem

Renal handling of water

The kidney regulates body water and sodium content in parallel to maintain body volume and osmolality (normally 285–295 mOsmol/kg) (see Chapter 12). The maximum urine osmolality is 1400 mOsmol/kg and, as 600 mOsmol of waste products must be excreted daily, the minimal daily urine volume is 600/1400 = 0.43 L. The kidney can produce urine with an osmolality that is higher or lower than that of plasma.

In the glomerulus, water and ions are freely filtered. As the filtrate moves along the tubules, ions are reabsorbed and water follows by osmosis. Water reabsorption is influenced by the water permeability of the tubular epithelium and the osmotic gradient across the epithelium. Water leaves and enters cells through aquaporin (**AQP**) water channels.

Proximal tubule

The proximal tubule is highly water permeable. As ions are reabsorbed, water follows by osmosis. This isotonic (or iso-osmotic) reabsorption reduces the filtrate volume, but does not alter its osmolality. Around 65% of the filtrate is reabsorbed, driven by active sodium transport.

Loop of Henle

The descending limb is permeable to water, but not ions, whereas the ascending limb (both thick and thin sections) is permeable to ions, but not water. Sodium and chloride are transported out of the thick ascending limb into the medullary interstitium. This raises the osmolality in the interstitium, which promotes water movement out of the descending limb. Within the loop, the transport of water and ions is separated with reabsorption of 25% of filtered sodium and chloride, but only 10% of filtered water. This produces a dilute urine and a hypertonic medullary interstitium. The movement of ions and water between the descending and ascending limbs creates a gradient of osmolality, which increases with depth in the medulla.

Distal tubules

The distal convoluted tubules have low water permeability and do not reabsorb water. However, reabsorption of ions further dilutes the tubular fluid.

Collecting system

The hypotonic urine passes down the collecting ducts, where water permeability is controlled by antidiuretic hormone (ADH or vasopressin).

• If the permeability of the collecting ducts is low, there is no water reabsorption, but sodium chloride reabsorption continues, which further dilutes the urine.

• If the permeability of the collecting ducts is high, water moves out of the hypotonic tubular fluid into the surrounding interstitium. In the cortical collecting duct, tubular fluid equilibrates with the cortical interstitium, which is at plasma osmolality. In the deeper medullary collecting duct, tubular fluid then equilibrates with the high osmolality of the medullary interstitium, producing a concentrated urine.

Overall, sodium and chloride transport out of the ascending limb of the loop of Henle creates a hypertonic medullary interstitium, which drives water reabsorption from the descending limb and the medullary collecting duct. All collecting ducts pass through the medulla, so even nephrons without long loops of Henle can benefit from the hypertonic medulla.

Role of urea

Although urea is passively reabsorbed in the proximal tubule, the nephron beyond is impermeable to urea up to the inner medullary collecting duct. As water is removed along the nephron, tubular urea concentration rises. In the inner medullary collecting duct, urea is passively reabsorbed by urea transporters (especially **UT-A1 and A3**) which are activated by vasopressin. This reabsorbed urea accounts for half of the medullary interstitial osmolality that drives water reabsorption from the descending limb and medullary collecting duct.

Vasa recta and counter-current exchange

If the medulla had normal blood capillaries, the interstitium would equilibrate with plasma. However, the only blood vessels supplying the medulla are the paired descending and ascending vessels called the vasa recta, which function as counter-current exchangers. As the vessels descend into the medulla, water diffuses out and solutes into the vessels. As the vessels ascend out of the medulla, water diffuses back in and solutes out of the vessels. The result is no net change in medullary water and solute content—the medullary osmolality therefore stays high. The vasa recta contain **UT-B** urea transporters that help to maintain medullary urea concentrations.

Vasopressin and water regulation

Vasopressin is a nine-amino-acid peptide made in the supraoptic and paraventricular nuclei of the hypothalamus. It is packaged into granules, which pass down axons to the posterior pituitary and are released by exocytosis. Osmoreceptors in the hypothalamus detect a rise in plasma osmolality above 280 mOsmol/kg and trigger vasopressin release. Other stimuli to vasopressin secretion include volume depletion, angiotensin II, hypoxia, hypercapnia, epinephrine (adrenaline), cortisol, sex steroids, pain, trauma, temperature, and psychogenic stimuli.

Vasopressin binds V_2 receptors on collecting duct cells. This stimulates adenyl cyclase, raising cAMP levels and causing intracellular vesicles to fuse with the apical membrane. In their membrane, these vesicles contain water channels, especially the 29-kDa aquaporin protein, **AQP2**. Vasopressin also binds to V_1 receptors on vascular smooth muscle, causing vasoconstriction and enhancing the effect of aldosterone on sodium reabsorption in the distal tubule. **AQP1**, a related protein in erythrocytes, forms hourglass-shaped water channels from membrane-spanning a helices. Amino acids in the narrow central part form a narrow channel that allows only water molecules to pass through.

12 Regulation of body sodium and body water

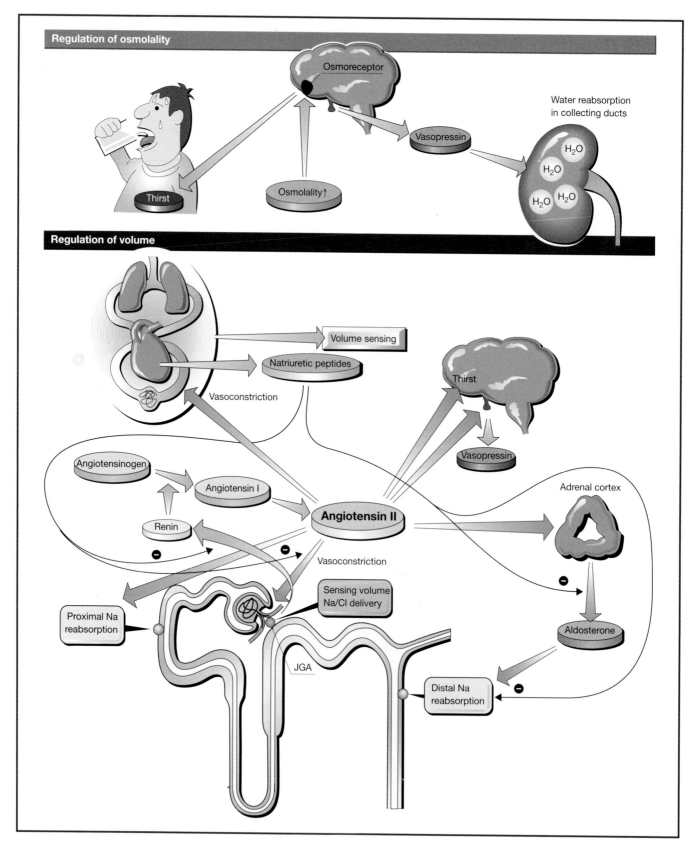

Total body volume reflects total body water content. The body senses osmolality and body volume, and regulates them by altering water and sodium content, respectively. Water can be moved only by osmosis and, as the major osmotically active extracellular ions are sodium salts, sodium and water regulation are tightly linked. The body directly controls the osmolality and volume of the intravascular extracellular fluid and this influences the osmolality and volumes of the other compartments.

Body water exists in the extracellular and intracellular compartments. The extracellular compartment consists of the intravascular and extravascular spaces, which are in approximate equilibrium. Sodium salts account for around 280 of the total 290 mOsmol/kg H_2O in the extracellular fluid. As sodium is actively pumped out of cells, sodium salts account for only 40 of the total 290 mOsmol/kg H_2O in the intracellular fluid.

Regulation of osmolality

Unless there is a massive volume change, such as an acute bleed, osmolality is usually maintained at the expense of volume changes. All body compartments are in approximate osmotic equilibrium, and there is only one set of osmoreceptors in the anterior hypothalamus, near the supraoptic nuclei. *The osmoreceptors control water intake by altering thirst and control renal water excretion by altering vasopressin release.*

Changes in sodium concentration influence osmolality. For example, salt ingestion raises plasma osmolality, provoking thirst and reducing renal water excretion. This increases body volume and reduces salt concentration and osmolality, but it does not alter the amount of salt present. Thus, osmoregulation controls plasma sodium concentration by altering the water balance, but it does not control body sodium content.

Regulation of volume

If the body sodium content is altered, the osmoregulatory system adjusts water balance and therefore the body volume to maintain normal osmolality. Therefore, body volume can be controlled by altering body sodium content. The kidney controls sodium excretion and therefore body volume. Body volume sensing is complex and there are multiple volume receptors. This input is integrated by the nervous system to produce a coordinated neural and endocrine response that regulates renal sodium excretion.

Sensing body volume

Baroreceptors respond to vascular stretch. **High-pressure arterial stretch receptors** detect low perfusion pressure, usually when intravascular volume is too low. **Low-pressure venous stretch receptors** detect whether intravascular volume is too high. Many receptors detect circulatory pressure, including atrial stretch receptors, the carotid baroreceptors, the juxtaglomerular apparatus, and various tissue mechanoreceptors. Many of these receptors have neural links to the hypothalamus and medulla.

Control of renal sodium excretion

Angiotensin II binds to AT1-receptors in the proximal tubule, activating the phosphoinositol secondary messenger system. This promotes apical Na^+/H^+ exchange and therefore sodium reabsorption. Angiotensin II also causes thirst and stimulates aldosterone production, vasopressin release, and renal and systemic vasoconstriction. Renin is released when the total body sodium falls. The stimulus is a fall in circulatory volume, which increases renal sympathetic nerve activity (mediated by β-adrenergic receptors), reduces afferent arteriolar tension, and reduces sodium chloride delivery to the macula densa.

Aldosterone diffuses into the principal cells of the collecting duct and binds to type 1 steroid receptors in the cytosol. This complex then migrates into the nucleus, promoting transcription of new apical sodium channels and basolateral Na^+/K^+ ATPases. These changes increase sodium reabsorption. Aldosterone is mainly regulated by the renin–angiotensin II system.

Natriuretic peptides. Atrial natriuretic peptide (ANP) is released from atrial cells on atrial distention and is also produced in collecting duct cells. It binds NPR-A receptors on collecting duct cells and acts via cGMP to inactivate apical sodium channels, so reducing sodium reabsorption. It also inhibits aldosterone release and renin production and increases the glomerular filtration rate by dilating afferent arterioles. BNP has similar effects.

Vasopressin (ADH or AVP) enhances water reabsorption in the collecting ducts (see Chapter 11). Prostaglandins produced in the medulla, especially PGE2, enhance sodium and water excretion and are vasodilators.

Dopamine is secreted in the proximal tubule and reduces sodium reabsorption by inhibiting Na^+/H^+ exchange. This effect is mediated by DA_1-receptors which activate adenyl cyclase; it is opposite to that of angiotensin II and α-adrenergic agonists. Dopamine is also a vasodilator.

α-Adrenergic agonists act via G proteins to enhance Na^+/H^+ exchange and increase sodium reabsorption in the proximal tubule.

Extracellular fluid volume directly influences sodium excretion. Proximal tubule sodium and chloride reabsorption requires the ultimate removal of these ions from the lateral intercellular spaces. If the extracellular fluid volume is increased, capillary hydrostatic pressure rises and plasma proteins are diluted, reducing the capillary osmotic pressure. These changes reduce salt and water uptake from the interspace between tubular cells, promoting sodium and water excretion and thus reducing the extracellular fluid volume.

13 Disorders of sodium and water metabolism

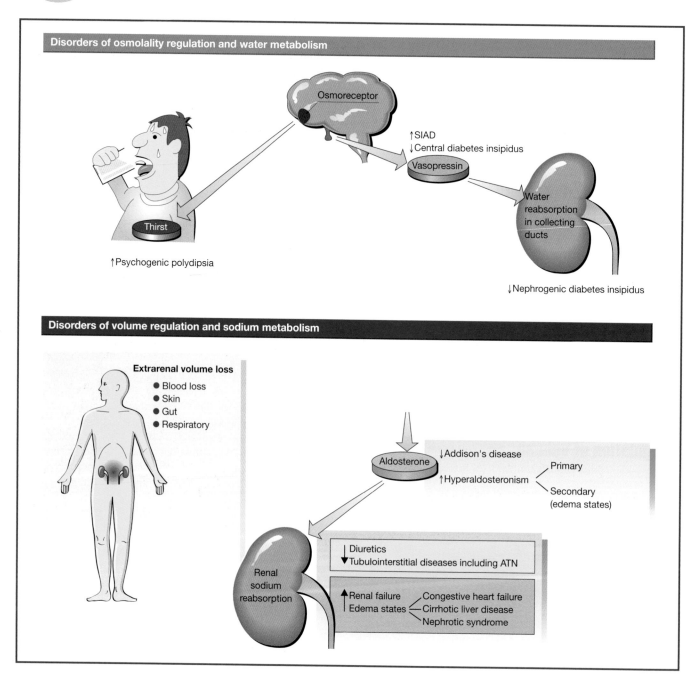

Disorders of osmolality regulation and water metabolism

Osmoreceptor

↑SIAD
↓Central diabetes insipidus

Vasopressin

Water reabsorption in collecting ducts

Thirst

↑Psychogenic polydipsia

↓Nephrogenic diabetes insipidus

Disorders of volume regulation and sodium metabolism

Extrarenal volume loss
- Blood loss
- Skin
- Gut
- Respiratory

Aldosterone

↓Addison's disease

↑Hyperaldosteronism — Primary
— Secondary (edema states)

↓Diuretics
↓Tubulointerstitial diseases including ATN

↑Renal failure — Congestive heart failure
Edema states — Cirrhotic liver disease
— Nephrotic syndrome

Renal sodium reabsorption

Disordered regulation of body volume or osmolality causes changes in body sodium or water content, respectively. Depending on the ratio of these changes, hyponatremia or hypernatremia can occur, with or without a change in body volume. Generally, hyponatremia and hypernatremia reflect hypoosmolality and hyperosmolality, respectively. To diagnose the cause of disordered sodium or water metabolism, try to evaluate body volume and osmolality.

Disordered water metabolism arises when *osmoregulation* is defective, resulting in too much or too little body water relative to the amount of body solute. The main solute is sodium, so too much water causes hyponatremia and too little causes hypernatremia. **Disordered sodium metabolism** arises when *volume regulation* is defective and there is inappropriate sodium retention or loss, causing the body volume to be too high or too low. **Mixed disorders** with abnormal volume and osmolality are common and alter both body sodium and water content.

The Renal System at a Glance, Fourth Edition. Chris O'Callaghan. © 2017 John Wiley & Sons, Ltd. Published 2017 by John Wiley & Sons, Ltd.
Companion website: www.ataglanceseries.com/renalsystem

Diagnosis is often difficult because initial pathological changes are altered by compensatory mechanisms. Loss of isotonic salt solution from the gut, for example, causes hypovolemia and this triggers thirst. However, if the patient then ingests water without salt, hyponatremia will result. Most disorders of solute loss cause some secondary water retention due to vasopressin secretion and so can cause hypo-osmolality. Extrarenal sodium or water loss can occur in body fluids such as blood, sweat, or gut secretions, especially diarrhea.

Disorders of water metabolism and osmolality control

Inadequate vasopressin action causes diabetes insipidus, whereas excess vasopressin action causes the syndrome of inappropriate diuresis (SIAD). Plasma hypo-osmolality normally suppresses vasopressin secretion and the minimum urine osmolality that can be produced is around 50 mOsmol/kg H_2O. A urine concentration of 800 mOsmol/kg H_2O is proof of normal vasopressin action.

Diabetes insipidus

Central diabetes insipidus occurs when the pituitary gland does not release enough vasopressin. It can arise if the pituitary or hypothalamus is damaged, particularly by trauma or a brain tumor.

Nephrogenic diabetes insipidus occurs when the kidney fails to respond to vasopressin. Causes include mutations in the V2 vasopressin receptor or the AQP2 channel, hypokalemia, hypercalcemia, and drugs, such as lithium, amphotericin, or gentamicin. Clinically, there is polyuria and polydipsia. Plasma osmolality and sodium are high and urine osmolality and sodium are low. Polydipsia and the high salt intake in Western diets often maintain a normal plasma sodium and body volume despite the urinary losses. However, water deprivation fails to increase urine osmolality as it should.

In nephrogenic diabetes insipidus, vasopressin levels are high and there is no response to synthetic vasopressin. In central diabetes insipidus, vasopressin levels are low and synthetic vasopressin causes a rise in urine osmolality. Intranasal desmopressin (DDAVP), a vasopressin agonist, is therefore used as therapy for central diabetes insipidus.

Syndrome of inappropriate diuresis (SIAD) or syndrome of inappropriate vasopressin (ADH) secretion (SIADH)

Inappropriately high vasopressin levels cause excess water reabsorption by the kidney. This causes low plasma osmolality and low plasma sodium concentration. Urine is inappropriately concentrated for the low plasma osmolality. Causes include the stress-induced vasopressin secretion that can occur postoperatively and with lung cancers, especially the small cell type, which can secrete vasopressin. Treatment is by restriction of water intake because even if there is excess vasopressin, the kidney continues to excrete some water and will eventually eliminate the excess water. Vaptans, such as tolvaptan, are antagonists of the V2 vasopressin receptor and can be used to treat SIAD. Demeclocycline causes nephrogenic diabetes insipidus and is sometimes used to treat SIAD. SIAD is the same as SIADH.

Psychogenic polydipsia

Massive abnormal water intake as a result of psychiatric disturbance can cause hypo-osmolality if water intake exceeds the capacity for its excretion.

Disorders of the volume regulatory mechanism and sodium metabolism

Inappropriate body volume control can occur if there is a primary abnormality of renal sodium handling. It can also occur when the kidney is normal, if there is an abnormality affecting the volume-sensing system, which drives inappropriate renal sodium handling.

Excess sodium excretion

Addison's disease is caused by destruction of the adrenal glands, usually by an autoimmune process or tuberculosis. As sodium reabsorption in the distal tubule is promoted by aldosterone, a deficiency of this hormone causes hyponatremia. Hyperkalemia also occurs because potassium secretion is mechanistically linked to sodium reabsorption in the distal tubule (see Chapter 29). The excess sodium excretion causes hypovolemia. Glucocorticoid deficiency, if present, may also cause hypoglycemia. There may be generalized pigmentation probably caused by the melanocyte-stimulating side effects of excess adrenocorticotrophic hormone (ACTH) produced by the pituitary, in an attempt to drive the adrenal gland. Autoimmune vitiligo can also occur. Treatment is with mineralocorticoid and glucocorticoid replacement.

Diuretics. These cause excess renal sodium excretion.

Intrinsic renal disease can cause renal salt wasting. Causes include tubulointerstitial disease because of its effects on tubular function and specific hereditary tubular conditions that affect renal salt handling (see Chapter 30).

Disorders causing inadequate sodium excretion

Excess aldosterone, whatever its cause, promotes excessive sodium reabsorption and enhanced potassium secretion in the distal tubule, causing hypernatremia and hypokalemia. Thirst is triggered, often causing polydipsia. Primary hyperaldosteronism is usually caused by an adrenal tumor or hyperplasia. Typically, plasma aldosterone levels are high and plasma renin levels are low.

Renal failure ultimately reduces the ability of the kidney to excrete sodium or indeed other electrolytes.

The edema syndromes (congestive heart failure, cirrhotic liver disease, and nephrotic syndrome) display an erroneously perceived reduction in body volume, promoting both sodium and water conservation (see Chapter 15).

14 Hyponatremia and hypernatremia

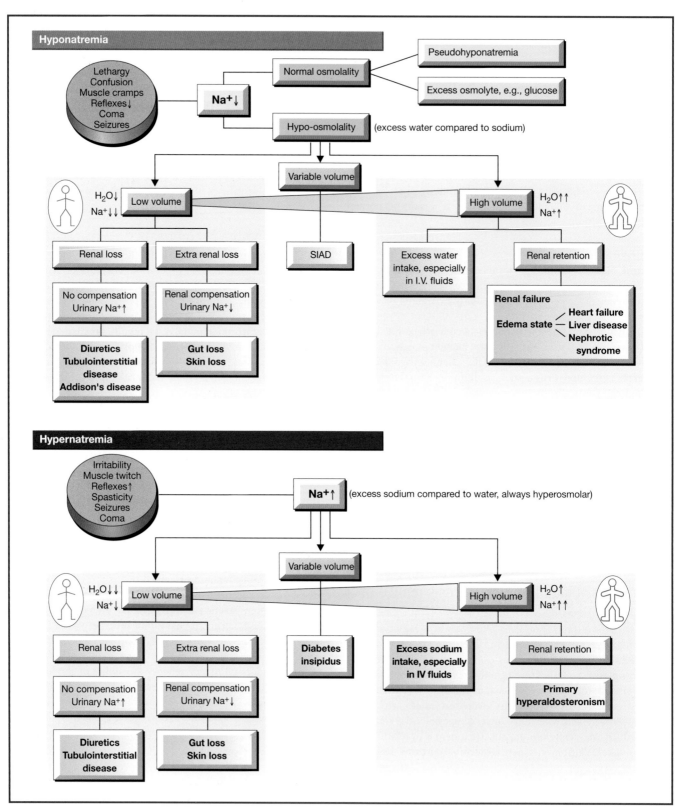

Hyponatremia

Lethargy
Confusion
Muscle cramps
Reflexes↓
Coma
Seizures

Na+↓

Normal osmolality
- Pseudohyponatremia
- Excess osmolyte, e.g., glucose

Hypo-osmolality (excess water compared to sodium)

Variable volume

H₂O↓ Na+↓↓ — Low volume

High volume — H₂O↑↑ Na+↑

- Renal loss
  - No compensation Urinary Na+↑
    - **Diuretics Tubulointerstitial disease Addison's disease**
- Extra renal loss
  - Renal compensation Urinary Na+↓
    - **Gut loss Skin loss**

SIAD

Excess water intake, especially in I.V. fluids

Renal retention
- **Renal failure**
- **Edema state** — **Heart failure Liver disease Nephrotic syndrome**

Hypernatremia

Irritability
Muscle twitch
Reflexes↑
Spasticity
Seizures
Coma

Na+↑ (excess sodium compared to water, always hyperosmolar)

Variable volume

H₂O↓↓ Na+↓ — Low volume

High volume — H₂O↑ Na+↑↑

- Renal loss
  - No compensation Urinary Na+↑
    - **Diuretics Tubulointerstitial disease**
- Extra renal loss
  - Renal compensation Urinary Na+↓
    - **Gut loss Skin loss**

Diabetes insipidus

Excess sodium intake, especially in IV fluids

Renal retention
- **Primary hyperaldosteronism**

The Renal System at a Glance, Fourth Edition. Chris O'Callaghan. © 2017 John Wiley & Sons, Ltd. Published 2017 by John Wiley & Sons, Ltd.
Companion website: www.ataglanceseries.com/renalsystem

Abnormal plasma sodium concentration indicates an imbalance between the amount of sodium and water in the body. Hyponatremia is usually associated with hypo-osmolality and hypernatremia with hyperosmolality. Plasma and extravascular extracellular fluids are in equilibrium, so their sodium concentrations are the same. Sodium is the major extracellular osmolyte and changes in sodium concentration cause osmotic movement of water into or out of cells. This can impair cellular function, especially in the nervous system. Acute changes cause more severe symptoms than chronic changes. With chronic changes, the cells reduce the osmotic effect on them by altering intracellular osmolality. They do this by altering intracellular concentrations of ions and of urea and amino acids.

To assess hyponatremia or hypernatremia, evaluate body volume and consider all routes of fluid or electrolyte loss and gain. It can be helpful to establish whether the kidneys are acting appropriately to compensate for the sodium abnormality or acting inappropriately to exacerbate the changes. This is determined by assessing whether the urine sodium concentration is appropriate for the body volume, plasma sodium concentration, and osmolality.

Hyponatremia

Hyponatremia always reflects hypo-osmolality unless there is pseudohyponatremia or an excess of another osmolyte in the plasma (e.g., an excess of glucose triggers a fall in plasma sodium to maintain normal osmolality). Both these situations are easily diagnosed because measured plasma osmolality is normal. Pseudohyponatremia occurs when there is excess protein or lipid in the plasma. Although the amount of sodium in each liter of plasma water is normal, the amount of water in each liter of total plasma is reduced because part of that volume of plasma is made up of the excess protein or lipid. Pseudohyponatremia is not a problem with modern ion-specific electrodes, which directly measure the sodium concentration in the aqueous phase.

True hyponatremia usually indicates excess water retention in relation to sodium. Water intake exceeds water excretion. Apart from urine, body fluids are not usually hypertonic, so their loss does not cause hyponatremia directly. However, sodium and water loss in body fluids causes hypovolemia, which triggers nonosmotic vasopressin secretion. Hyponatremia then follows if volume replacement is with water, which dilutes the body sodium and is retained as a result of the vasopressin.

In the absence of diuretics and kidney disease, urine osmolality <100 mOsm/kg indicates suppression of vasopressin release due to excess drinking with an appropriately dilute urine. Urine osmolality >100 mOsm/kg indicates vasopressin activity. In this context, a urine sodium concentration <30 mmol/L indicates renal sodium conservation which may be appropriate in hypovolemia (e.g., with diarrhea and vomiting) or inappropriate with fluid overload in an edema state (Chapter 15) (e.g., heart failure). Conversely, with a urine osmolality of >100 mOsmol/kg, a urine sodium concentration of >30 mmol/L indicates renal sodium loss which can indicate SIAD(H), adrenal insufficiency, a renal salt-wasting condition, diuretics or hypothyroidism.

Clinical features

Hyponatremia causes brain edema because water enters brain cells by osmosis. Mostly it is asymptomatic, but young and elderly people, menstruating women, and those with underlying neurological conditions or other metabolic disorders are more vulnerable to symptoms. Clinical manifestations are initially those of depressed function, including lethargy, confusion, agitation, muscle cramps, nausea, and reduced tendon reflexes. Ultimately, seizures and coma can occur, particularly when sodium levels fall below 120 mmol/L. Mortality from hyponatremia can be high, but it is dangerous to correct hyponatremia too rapidly, because this can cause neurological damage.

Treatment

The underlying cause should be corrected. If the body volume is high, treatment is restriction of fluid intake to reduce excess body water. Sometimes, diuretics can be useful, but they may exacerbate the hyponatremia. If body volume is low, the missing sodium and water should be replaced, usually with isotonic saline. Plasma sodium should be regularly checked to ensure that correction is not too rapid (aim for no more than 10–12 mmol/L per day or 18 mmol in 48 h). Specific antagonists of vasopressin known as vaptans may be useful in hyponatremia, principally when body volume is high or normal. Selective V2 receptor antagonists such as tolvaptan are not associated with the hypotension that could arise with nonselective vasopressin antagonists.

Hypernatremia

Hypernatremia usually results from a deficiency of body water relative to sodium, as happens in diabetes insipidus. Hypernatremia always causes hyperosmolality because sodium is the major extracellular ion. However, hyperosmolality can also result from excesses of other osmolytes, most commonly glucose in diabetes mellitus or urea in renal failure.

Most hypernatremia arises from unreplaced water loss, so the body volume is usually low. The body's main defense against hypernatremia is therefore thirst. Thirst is often inadequate in elderly people or sick patients with no access to oral fluids. Hypernatremia can also result from excess aldosterone, which causes excess sodium retention. Hypernatremia can occur if urine-concentrating mechanisms are inefficient and urine is dilute with low sodium content. This occurs in diabetes insipidus and tubulointerstitial disease, and with diuretic use.

Clinical features

Hyperosmolality causes brain cells to shrink as water leaves them by osmosis. Various neurological problems can occur, including tearing of cerebral vessels. Early clinical features are those of increased excitability, including irritability, muscle twitches, brisk reflexes, and spasticity. Ultimately, seizures and coma can occur. Children seem particularly vulnerable and mortality can be high.

Treatment

This includes correction of water deficits and prevention of ongoing loss, by correcting any underlying cause. Depending on the severity, replacement is with oral water or an intravenous 5% dextrose (glucose) solution (the dextrose is removed by metabolism). As with hyponatremia, plasma sodium should be regularly checked during treatment to ensure that correction is not too rapid (aim for 12 mmol/L per hour).

15 The edema states: sodium and water retention

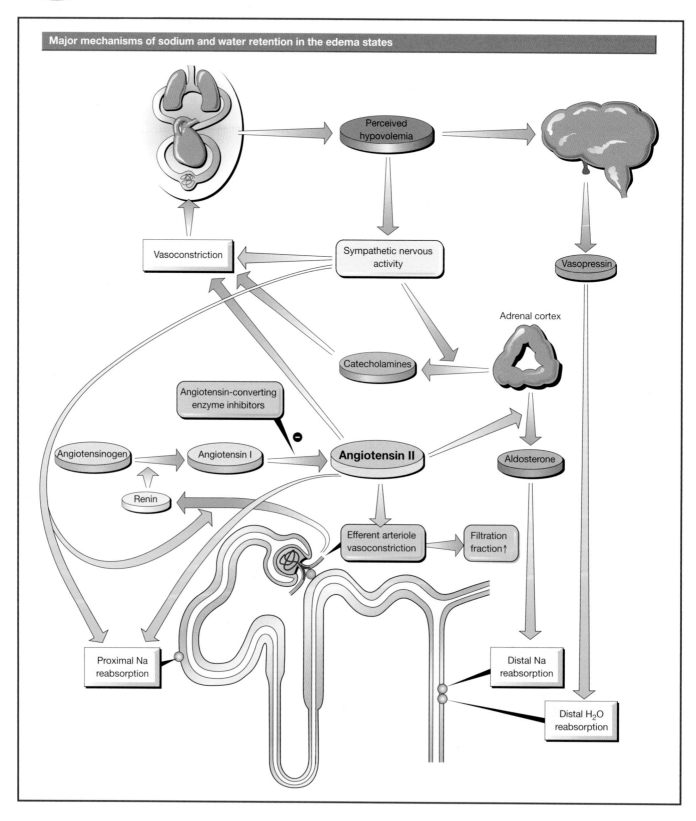

Major mechanisms of sodium and water retention in the edema states

Normally, the high hydrostatic pressure of arterial blood entering tissue capillary beds causes some fluid to filter through the capillary wall into the interstitial space. Toward the venous end of the capillary bed, hydrostatic pressure falls, and the loss of fluid results in a rise in the plasma osmolality as a result of plasma proteins. These changes promote fluid movement back into the blood. Changes in capillary hydrostatic or osmotic pressure can cause edema, the accumulation of excess fluid in the interstitium. Venous obstruction or hypervolemia raises hydrostatic pressure at the venous end of the capillary bed, which reduces interstitial fluid reabsorption. A low plasma protein concentration lowers the capillary osmotic pressure and reduces interstitial fluid reabsorption.

Generalized edema occurs only when the body volume is too high. This can happen in advanced renal failure because the kidneys cannot excrete enough sodium or water. However, the major causes are congestive heart failure, cirrhotic liver disease, and nephrotic syndrome. In these conditions, renal sodium-handling mechanisms are intact, but the kidney receives neuroendocrine signals that promote sodium and water retention. This occurs because the volume sensors perceive that the circulation is underfilled and drive a volume-conserving response similar to that during hemorrhage. This response includes enhanced sympathetic and catecholamine activity, enhanced renin–angiotensin II–aldosterone activity, and excess vasopressin secretion.

The afferent defect: perceived hypovolemia

Arterial baroreceptors are the dominant volume sensors, and monitor the stretching of arterial walls. In congestive heart failure, reduced cardiac output lowers the blood pressure, which stimulates arterial baroreceptors. In cirrhotic liver disease, a fall in systemic vascular resistance lowers the blood pressure and triggers arterial baroreceptors. Low vascular resistance is caused by splanchnic vasodilation and the development of multiple arteriovenous shunts, including spider nevi in the skin. The vasodilation may be caused by either raised nitric oxide levels or a failure of the diseased liver to degrade other vasoactive substances. The volume-conserving response in nephrotic syndrome is less clearly understood. One possibility is that heavy proteinuria lowers plasma protein levels, allowing fluid to leak into the interstitium. The reduced circulating volume would then trigger a volume-conserving response.

The efferent volume-conserving response

Increased *sympathetic activity* mediated by α-adrenergic receptors promotes sodium reabsorption in the proximal tubule and reduces renal blood flow by renal vasoconstriction. This vasoconstriction, and any fall in the blood pressure, lower afferent arteriolar pressure, in turn promoting renin secretion. Stimulation of β-adrenergic receptors also promotes renin release. A raised *angiotensin II* level causes further vasoconstriction and promotes proximal tubule sodium reabsorption. It also triggers *aldosterone* release, which increases distal tubular sodium reabsorption. The nonosmotic stimulation of *vasopressin* secretion promotes water retention and, if this is excessive in relation to the sodium retention, hyponatremia can occur. *Renal hemodynamics* may be relevant. A rise in the filtration fraction increases peritubular capillary osmotic pressure, which promotes water and sodium reabsorption.

Hepatorenal syndrome. In severe liver disease, the efferent response can occasionally produce such a powerful vasoconstrictive effect that the glomerular filtration rate falls rapidly and acute renal failure occurs.

Location of edema

Edema fluid collects in slack tissues that are low in the body. Here, gravity causes a high hydrostatic venous pressure, opposing interstitial fluid reabsorption. Clinically, edema may be detectable as pulmonary edema in the lungs or as peripheral edema around the ankles, sacrum, and scrotum. Excess fluid can also accumulate as effusions, such as pleural effusions or ascites. In liver cirrhosis, hepatic fibrosis causes postsinusoidal obstruction in the liver. This encourages fluid movement out of the liver and into the peritoneum as ascites.

Clinical features

High body volume usually raises the venous pressure, causing a high jugular venous pulse pressure. Outside the circulation, there is subcutaneous pitting edema – fluid moves away from a point where pressure is applied. Pulmonary edema can be heard with a stethoscope as fine inspiratory crackles.

Treatment

The primary disorder should be treated if possible. Edema may not need treatment unless it is impairing function. Initially, sodium restriction may be useful and water restriction is also appropriate if there is hyponatremia. Thiazide or loop **diuretics** promote sodium excretion and, if hypokalemia is a problem, potassium-sparing diuretics can be used. In heart failure, **angiotensin-converting enzyme inhibitors** are the first-line therapy because they block the vasoconstrictive and sodium-retaining actions of angiotensin II (as do angiotensin II receptor blockers). The ascites of cirrhotic liver disease dissipates slowly, and large volumes are often drained percutaneously. Diuretics are given concurrently to reduce the reaccumulation of fluid, and intravenous albumin can be used to promote the retention of fluid in the circulation. As many cirrhotic patients have substantial hyperaldosteronism, potassium depletion is common and **spironolactone** reduces potassium loss.

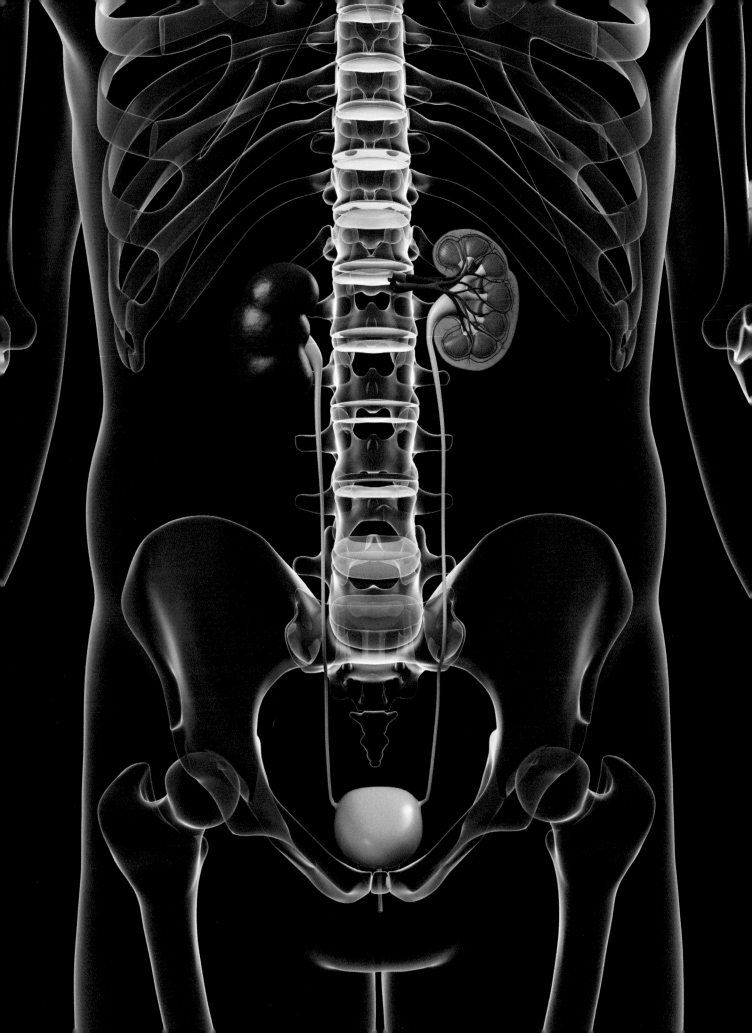

Potassium

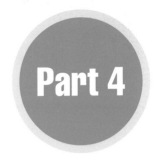

Part 4

Chapters

16 **Renal potassium handling** 38
17 **Regulation of potassium metabolism** 40
18 **Hypokalemia and hyperkalemia** 42

Don't forget to visit the companion website for this book
www.ataglanceseries.com/renalsystem

16 Renal potassium handling

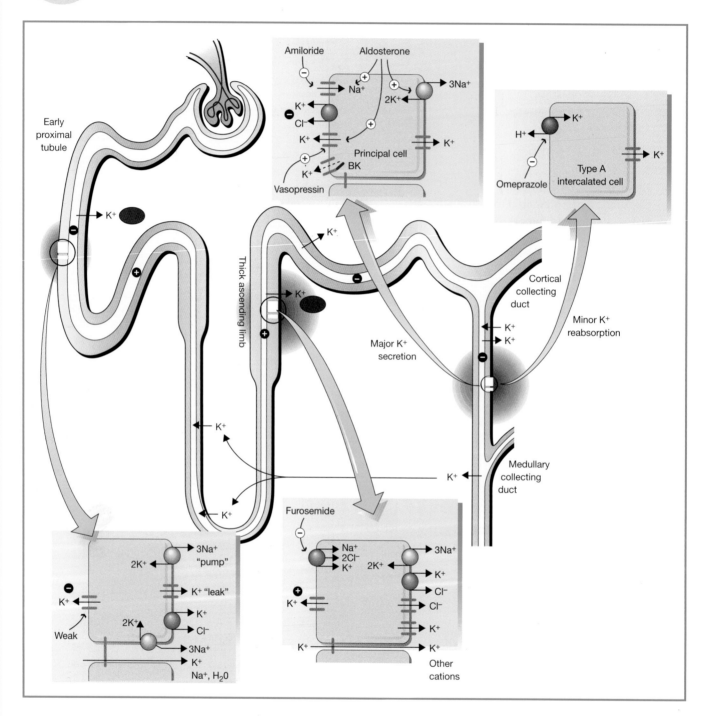

Potassium is the major intracellular cation. The potassium concentration inside cells is around 150 mmol/L, compared with around 4 mmol/L in extracellular fluid. The K^+ gradient across the cell membrane largely determines the electrical potential across that membrane. As this electrical potential influences the electrical excitability of tissues such as nerves and muscles, including the cardiac muscle, potassium levels must be precisely controlled within safe limits.

The average daily intake of potassium in the diet is around 40–120 mmol, but the kidneys filter around 800 mmol each day. To maintain potassium balance, the kidney therefore excretes only 5–15% of the filtered potassium. Potassium, like sodium, is freely filtered in the glomerulus, but is handled quite differently in the tubules. Sodium ions are reabsorbed throughout the nephron, and any sodium that is excreted is simply that which has not been reabsorbed. In contrast, almost all the filtered potassium is reabsorbed before the filtrate reaches the collecting tubules. Potassium that is to be excreted is then secreted into the collecting duct.

Only 2% of the total body potassium is outside cells in the extracellular fluid and, in order to maintain appropriate intracellular potassium concentrations, all cells use a **pump–leak** mechanism. This consists of the Na^+/K^+ ATPase pump, which actively transports potassium into the cell, balanced by various channels, which allow potassium to leak out of the cell. Intracellular potassium can be controlled by changing the activity of the pump or by altering the number or the permeability of the potassium channels. In tubular cells, the cell membrane is divided into apical and basolateral portions, each of which has different populations of pumps and channels. This allows the pump–leak system to be used to transport potassium across the tubular epithelium. As with sodium handling, the major driving force behind potassium movement is the Na^+/K^+ ATPase.

Potassium channels in the kidney

All cell types have potassium channels, and there are different types of potassium channels, even within the kidney. The basic structure of all K^+ channels is a tetramer of membrane-spanning subunits with a central pore. The **ROMK channel** is present in all nephron segments except the proximal tubule and is the key secretory channel in the principal cells of the cortical collecting ducts. The channels are generally open, and are said to be inwardly rectifying because they favor potassium flow out of the cell. In the distal nephron apical **BK channels** play a role in potassium secretion and consist of a pore-forming alpha unit and a regulatory beta unit. BK channels are generally closed, but high flow rates trigger a rise in intracellular calcium that causes the channels to open.

Potassium handling along the nephron

Proximal tubule

Of the filtered potassium ions, 65% are reabsorbed in the proximal tubule. No specific potassium channels for this reabsorption have been identified. Potassium reabsorption is tightly linked to that of sodium and water, with similar proportions of the filtered sodium, water, and potassium being reabsorbed in this segment. The reabsorption of sodium drives that of water, which may carry some potassium with it. The potassium gradient resulting from the reabsorption of water from the tubular lumen drives the paracellular reabsorption of potassium and may be enhanced by the removal of potassium from the paracellular space via the Na^+/K^+ ATPase. In the later proximal tubule, the positive potential in the lumen also drives potassium reabsorption through the paracellular route.

Loop of Henle

Thin segments

Some potassium moves into the filtrate in the thin descending limb of the loop of Henle, but this is counterbalanced by movement of potassium out of the loop and into the medullary collecting ducts. The net result is some recycling of this potassium across the medullary interstitium.

Thick ascending limb

Around 30% of the filtered potassium is reabsorbed in the thick ascending limb of the loop of Henle. As in the proximal tubule, this potassium reabsorption is linked to sodium reabsorption. This is mediated by the NKCC2 transporter, but there is also significant paracellular reabsorption, encouraged by the positive potential in the tubular lumen.

Distal tubule

The distal tubule can reabsorb more potassium and 95% of the filtered potassium is reabsorbed in a sodium-dependent fashion before the filtrate reaches the collecting ducts.

Collecting tubule and ducts

The principal cells secrete potassium whereas the intercalated cells reabsorb potassium. Generally, potassium secretion far outweighs its reabsorption in this part of the nephron. The regulation of potassium excretion occurs here and is mainly the result of changes in potassium secretion by the principal cells, rather than changes in potassium reabsorption by the intercalated cells.

- **Principal cells.** The Na^+/K^+ ATPase drives potassium secretion in principal cells by pumping potassium into the cells at the basolateral surface. The basolateral surface is not very permeable to potassium, but at the apical surface, potassium ions can leave the cell through potassium channels or in co-transport with chloride via **KCC** channels. The negative potential in the tubular lumen due to sodium reabsorption also promotes potassium secretion. As potassium secretion is occurring down a concentration gradient, it can continue only if the concentration of potassium in the filtrate is kept low. A high flow rate carries away the secreted potassium and, *the higher the flow rate, the greater the amount of potassium that can be secreted and excreted.* In addition, as flow rates increase, BK channels open to increase the flow of potassium into the tubules.
- **Type A intercalated cells.** The reabsorption of potassium by the intercalated cells is driven by the apical H^+/K^+ ATPase which actively pumps potassium into the cell. Potassium ions leave the cells through the basolateral potassium channels and so are reabsorbed.

Medullary collecting ducts

There is some potassium reabsorption in the medullary collecting ducts, but potassium reaching the medullary interstitium is largely recycled by reabsorption into the thin descending loop of Henle.

17 Regulation of potassium metabolism

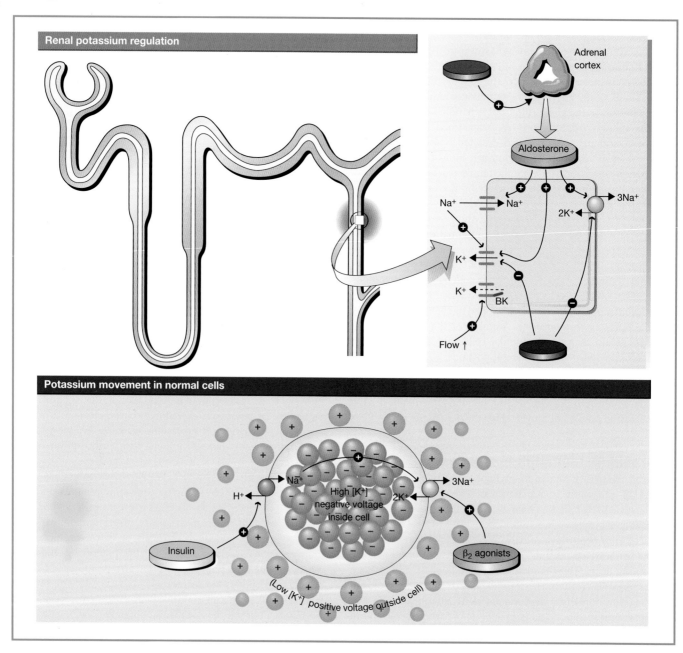

Renal potassium regulation

Potassium movement in normal cells

Potassium shifts across the cell membrane

The Na$^+$/K$^+$ ATPase pumps potassium into cells, and the slow leak of K$^+$ out of cells through K$^+$ channels generates a negative potential inside all cells relative to the outside. This is the resting membrane potential from which the action potential starts in excitable cells. When extracellular potassium falls, the potassium gradient across the cell membrane is increased. In cardiac cells, this slows repolarization, which slows the heart rate and keeps the cells nearer to their threshold for firing for longer than usual. During this slower repolarization, they are easily excited through triggering of sodium channels. Hypokalemia can therefore cause enhanced neuronal excitability and cardiac dysrhythmias. Conversely, a rise in extracellular potassium reduces the potassium gradient, which inactivates sodium channels and tends to make membranes less excitable, but vulnerable to fibrillation.

In both cases, the nature of any symptoms depends to some extent on the duration of the potassium abnormality and the rate of its development. Intracellular potassium levels do tend to change to compensate for the extracellular fluctuation. Chronic hypokalemia causes a shift of potassium out of the cells and chronic hyperkalemia a shift into them.

Influences on potassium movements across cell membranes

Insulin promotes Na$^+$/H$^+$ exchange across cell membranes, and the rise in intracellular sodium promotes K$^+$ entry by the

The Renal System at a Glance, Fourth Edition. Chris O'Callaghan. © 2017 John Wiley & Sons, Ltd. Published 2017 by John Wiley & Sons, Ltd.
Companion website: www.ataglanceseries.com/renalsystem

Na$^+$/K$^+$ ATPase. Postprandial insulin release reduces the impact on plasma potassium of gut absorption of potassium after a meal.

β_2-*Adrenergic agonists* activate the Na$^+$/K$^+$ ATPase, so β blockade can increase plasma potassium whereas β agonists can reduce it. Muscle cells release potassium during exercise leading to a rise in plasma potassium. However, catecholamine production during exercise promotes cellular potassium uptake and helps reduce the rise in plasma potassium.

pH. When H$^+$ ions enter the cells, they can displace K$^+$, so acidosis can raise plasma K$^+$ levels.

Thyroid hormones promote Na$^+$/K$^+$ ATPase synthesis and this can cause hypokalemia.

Renal potassium handling

The kidney and adrenal cortex regulate potassium levels, so abnormal potassium levels generally reflect renal or adrenal abnormalities. Homeostatic control of body potassium content is achieved by altering renal potassium handling. Although potassium reabsorption occurs mainly in the proximal tubule and thick ascending limb of the loop of Henle, the final potassium content of urine is controlled by potassium secretion in the cortical collecting duct.

The ROMK potassium channels in the cortical collecting duct are freely open for potassium movement, but movement of potassium into the filtrate requires a negative voltage in the lumen. This negative potential is generated by reabsorption of Na+ through the ENaC channel, which is controlled by aldosterone. Thus, sodium reabsorption promotes potassium secretion by making the tubule lumen negatively charged. When sodium reabsorption is inhibited, as with amiloride, potassium secretion is less efficient. Conversely, enhanced delivery of sodium to the distal tubule promotes potassium secretion.

Control of renal potassium excretion

Renal potassium excretion increases in parallel with plasma potassium concentration. An increase in the potassium concentration of extracellular fluid increases the activity of the Na$^+$/K$^+$ ATPase at the basolateral surface of the principal cells of the cortical collecting ducts; this drives potassium secretion into the lumen. The reverse occurs when the plasma concentration falls. In addition, several other factors play important roles.

Aldosterone

A rise in the potassium concentration in the extracellular fluid of the adrenal cortex directly stimulates aldosterone release. In the cortical collecting duct, aldosterone promotes the synthesis of Na$^+$/K$^+$ ATPases and the insertion of more Na$^+$/K$^+$ ATPases into the basolateral membrane. Aldosterone also stimulates apical sodium and potassium channel activity, increasing sodium reabsorption and potassium secretion (see Chapters 10 and 16).

pH changes

Potassium secretion is reduced in acute acidosis and increased in acute alkalosis. A higher pH increases the apical potassium channel activity and the basolateral Na$^+$/K$^+$ ATPase activity – both changes that promote potassium secretion. With chronic changes in pH, compensatory changes can occur, but chronic metabolic alkalosis is still usually associated with a low potassium level.

Flow rates

Increased flow rates in the collecting duct reduce potassium concentration in the lumen and, therefore, enhance potassium secretion. In addition, increased flow activates BK potassium channels causing increased potassium secretion (see Chapter 16). BK channel activation may arise from bending of cilia on the cells and subsequent rises in intracellular calcium. Increased flow also activates ENaC channels which will promote sodium reabsorption and so potassium secretion.

Sodium delivery

If the sodium delivery to the collecting duct falls, there is less sodium reabsorption. This reduces sodium levels in principal cells, reducing the activity of the Na$^+$/K$^+$ ATPase, which lowers intracellular potassium levels and reduces the gradient for potassium secretion. Also, as described above, sodium reabsorption promotes the lumen-negative potential difference, which drives potassium secretion.

Vasopressin

Vasopressin reduces urinary flow rates that would reduce potassium secretion. However, it also stimulates apical potassium channel activity, which helps maintain normal potassium secretion.

Magnesium

Intracellular magnesium can bind and block the pore of the ROMK channels, thus reducing potassium secretion into the tubules. Magnesium deficiency lowers the intracellular magnesium concentration in the tubular cells, which reduces this inhibitory effect and so allows more potassium to be secreted into the tubules. Therefore, magnesium deficiency can cause hypokalemia. Hypokalemia associated with magnesium deficiency can be difficult to treat until magnesium levels have been corrected.

Drugs affecting potassium excretion

The most important drugs affecting potassium excretion are diuretics, which increase urinary flow rates. The rise in the flow rate in the collecting ducts is the main factor in diuretic-induced potassium loss. Individual drugs have additional effects.

Thiazide diuretics reduce sodium and chloride reabsorption in the distal tubule. As potassium reabsorption in the distal tubule depends on sodium reabsorption, there is reduced potassium reabsorption.

Furosemide and the other loop diuretics inhibit potassium reabsorption via the NKCC2 co-transporter.

Spironolactone antagonizes the effects of aldosterone and so reduces potassium secretion.

Amiloride blocks apical sodium entry into principal cells, reducing the concentration of intracellular sodium available for the Na$^+$/K$^+$ ATPase, which normally drives potassium secretion.

Integration with sodium and volume regulation

With fluid depletion the renin–angiotensin system is activated with production of angiotensin II and so of aldosterone. Angiotensin II acts via WNK4 to inhibit ROMK channels so there is no excessive potassium loss with volume depletion. Pure hyperkalemia triggers aldosterone production directly without angiotensin II. The hyperkalemia acts via WNK1 to inhibit NCC activity and promote ROMK activity and so aids aldosterone-driven potassium secretion without excess sodium retention.

18 Hypokalemia and hyperkalemia

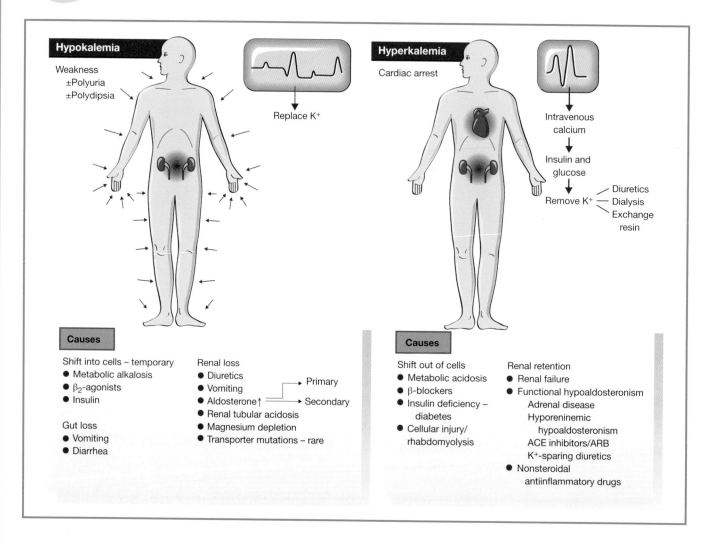

Abnormal plasma potassium levels can be life threatening. Potassium is the main determinant of the resting membrane potential of excitable cells, and disturbances of plasma potassium can cause cardiac dysrhythmias or arrest. The distinction between the electrocardiographic (ECG) abnormalities produced by hypokalemia and hyperkalemia is critical and may be lifesaving.

Hypokalemia

Hypokalemia usually reflects loss of potassium from the gut or kidney or, less commonly, a shift into the cells. In the kidneys, potassium loss can result from excess aldosterone or excess sodium delivery to the distal tubule, as can occur with loop or thiazide diuretic use. Excess aldosterone promotes sodium reabsorption and potassium secretion.

Causes

Loop diuretics, thiazide diuretics, and osmotic diuretics cause renal potassium excretion.

Hypokalemia associated with vomiting usually results from loss of potassium through the kidneys, rather than from the gut. Loss of acid gastric contents causes a metabolic alkalosis, which raises the plasma bicarbonate concentration and also the bicarbonate concentration in the filtrate. The excess sodium delivery to the distal tubule (as sodium bicarbonate) increases potassium secretion. There is often also volume depletion and aldosterone release, both of which further enhance potassium secretion.

Renal tubular acidoses can also cause hypokalemia (Chapter 24). In proximal renal tubular acidosis, excess sodium delivery to the distal tubule as sodium bicarbonate increases potassium secretion. In distal renal tubular acidosis, more potassium is excreted to maintain electroneutrality because sodium is reabsorbed in the distal tubule.

Other causes of hypokalemia include the following:
- Acute stress such as that of acute myocardial infarction. This causes a β_2-adrenergic-receptor-mediated shift of potassium into cells.
- Insulin excess or overdose.

The Renal System at a Glance, Fourth Edition. Chris O'Callaghan. © 2017 John Wiley & Sons, Ltd. Published 2017 by John Wiley & Sons, Ltd.
Companion website: www.ataglanceseries.com/renalsystem

• Magnesium depletion. This allows increased secretion of potassium through the ROMK channels resulting in hypokalemia (see Chapter 17). Magnesium may also lower cellular potassium levels probably by an effect on the Na$^+$/K$^+$ ATPase. Potassium deficiency is difficult to correct if magnesium is deficient.

• Drugs such as penicillins, aminoglycosides, and amphotericin can cause renal potassium loss.

• Mutations in the loop of Henle NKCC2 co-transporter, the distal tubule NCC NaCl co-transporter, or the collecting duct ENaC (see Chapter 30).

• Hypokalemic periodic paralysis is a rare autosomal dominant disorder characterized by periodic attacks of paralysis associated with hypokalemia.

Clinical features

Symptoms are unusual unless the potassium level is very low. There may be muscle weakness, constipation, or gut ileus. Polyuria and compensatory polydipsia can occur as a result of renal vasopressin (ADH) resistance. Hypokalemia predisposes to digoxin toxicity.

ECG changes

Hypokalemia increases automaticity and delays repolarization of cardiac cells. This predisposes the heart to dysrhythmias such as ectopic beats, atrioventricular block, and atrial and ventricular fibrillation. The classic changes are progressive lengthening of the P–R interval, S–T segment depression, flattening of the T waves, and an increase in the U wave.

Treatment

Potassium administration, usually as oral or intravenous potassium chloride, is the usual treatment. If metabolic alkalosis is present, potassium bicarbonate can be given. If the problem is caused by a diuretic, a potassium-sparing diuretic can be added.

Hyperkalemia

Hyperkalemia usually represents reduced urinary potassium secretion or, less commonly, acute release from cells or a failure to enter cells. Hyperkalemia does not persist unless there is impaired renal excretion. Remember that, if cells in a blood sample are hemolyzed, intracellular potassium has been released into the plasma and this can cause a spuriously elevated plasma potassium estimation.

Causes

Shifts out of cells. During metabolic acidosis, H$^+$ ions enter cells to be buffered and K$^+$ ions leave the cells to maintain electroneutrality. Insulin deficiency in diabetic ketoacidosis allows the net movement of potassium out of the cells. Rhabdomyolysis or tissue destruction, or lysis such as that caused by chemotherapy, can cause massive potassium loss from cells.

Failure of renal secretion. In renal failure, potassium accumulates because of the reduced number of nephrons capable of potassium excretion.

Other causes of hyperkalemia include the following:

• Trimethoprim and pentamidine therapy. Both can block potassium secretion in the collecting tubule.

• Hypoaldosteronism. The hyperkalemia can result from inadequate renin release, inadequate aldosterone release, or tubular resistance to aldosterone. Aldosterone normally stimulates tubular sodium reabsorption and potassium secretion. Hypoaldosteronism is usually caused by potassium-sparing diuretics or hyporeninemic hypoaldosteronism. The latter usually arises in diabetic nephropathy when there is a reduced glomerular filtration rate and reduced renin secretion.

• Angiotensin-converting enzyme inhibitors or angiotensin receptor blockers. These drugs reduce the aldosterone release that is normally promoted by angiotensin II and so reduce aldosterone-driven tubular potassium secretion.

• Pseudohypoaldosteronism. These syndromes are associated with a high potassium level but aldosterone levels are not raised. They are caused by inactivating mutations of the ENaC or WNK1 or WNK4 mutations which cause overactivity of the NCC sodium chloride co-transporter (see Chapter 30).

Clinical features

Symptoms, if present, include muscle weakness and cardiac dysrhythmias. The key cardiac dysrhythmia – ventricular fibrillation – causes cardiac arrest.

ECG changes

The typical ECG changes of hyperkalemia are loss of P waves, widening of the QRS complex, loss of the S–T segment, and tall-wide T waves. As the potassium level rises, the changes take on a sine wave appearance. The first change is the appearance of a narrowed, peaked T wave (this represents rapid repolarization); then the QRS widens into the T wave and the P wave is lost.

Treatment

The patient should be placed on a cardiac monitor. If there are ECG changes, urgent treatment is essential.

• Initially, calcium, given as calcium gluconate or calcium chloride, will antagonize the effects of potassium on the cardiac action potential, but this is short-lived.

• In the intermediate term, potassium can be shifted into cells by administering insulin, combined with glucose, to prevent hypoglycemia. β$_2$-agonists can also be used for this purpose. Administration of sodium bicarbonate produces a temporary alkalosis, which also promotes the intracellular movement of potassium.

• In the longer term, excess potassium must be removed from the body. Diuretics, such as furosemide, combined with hydration, encourage renal excretion. If renal function is severely impaired, dialysis or hemofiltration will remove potassium. Cation exchange resins such as sodium polystyrene sulfonate can be given orally or rectally and bind potassium in the gut, exchanging it for sodium. However their action is modest, relatively slow and they can cause severe constipation.

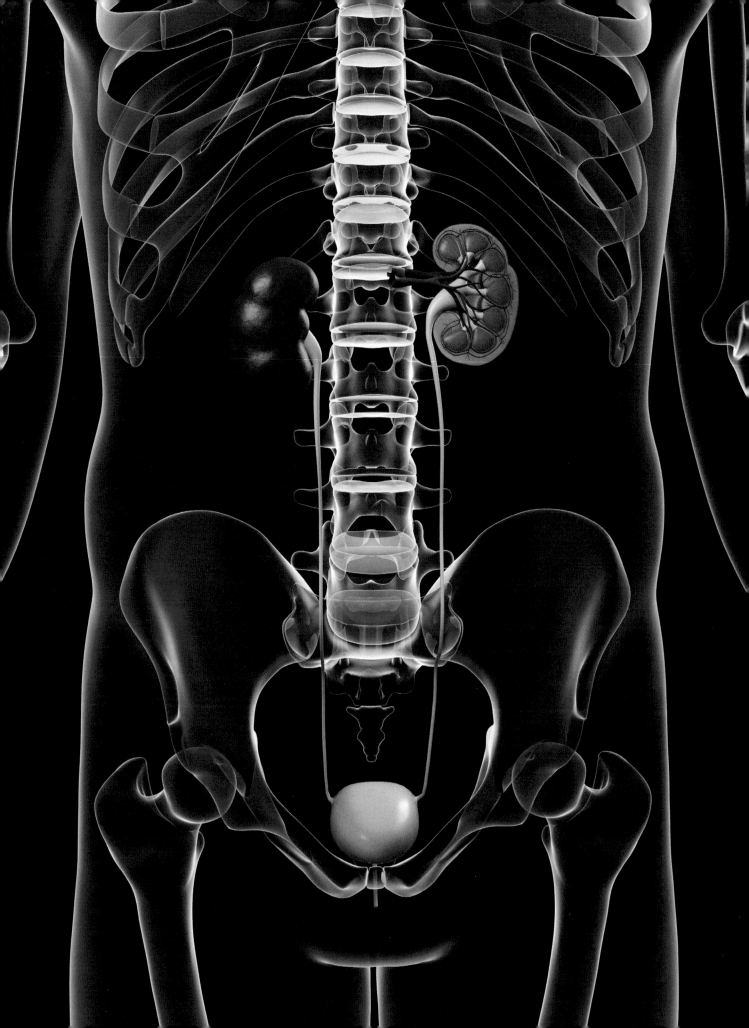

Acid-base

Part 5

Chapters

Don't forget to visit the companion website for this book
www.ataglanceseries.com/renalsystem

19 Renal acid-base and buffer concepts 46
20 Renal acid-base handling 48
21 Acid-base regulation and responses to acid-base disturbances 50
22 Clinical disorders of acid-base metabolism and metabolic acidosis 52
23 Metabolic alkalosis, respiratory acidosis, and respiratory alkalosis 54
24 Renal tubular acidosis 56

19 Renal acid-base and buffer concepts

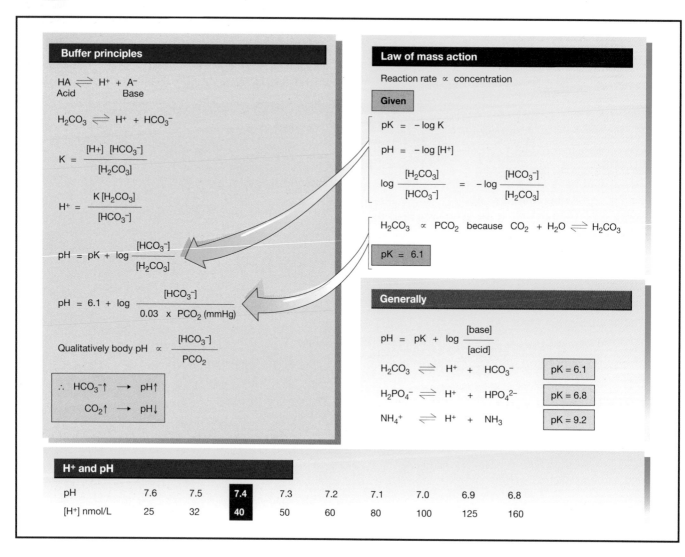

Buffer principles

$$HA \rightleftharpoons H^+ + A^-$$
$$\text{Acid} \qquad\quad \text{Base}$$

$$H_2CO_3 \rightleftharpoons H^+ + HCO_3^-$$

$$K = \frac{[H^+]\,[HCO_3^-]}{[H_2CO_3]}$$

$$H^+ = \frac{K\,[H_2CO_3]}{[HCO_3^-]}$$

$$pH = pK + \log \frac{[HCO_3^-]}{[H_2CO_3]}$$

$$pH = 6.1 + \log \frac{[HCO_3^-]}{0.03 \times PCO_2\ (mmHg)}$$

Qualitatively body pH $\propto \dfrac{[HCO_3^-]}{PCO_2}$

$$\therefore\ HCO_3^- \uparrow \longrightarrow pH \uparrow$$
$$CO_2 \uparrow \longrightarrow pH \downarrow$$

Law of mass action

Reaction rate $\propto$ concentration

Given

$$pK = -\log K$$

$$pH = -\log [H^+]$$

$$\log \frac{[H_2CO_3]}{[HCO_3^-]} = -\log \frac{[HCO_3^-]}{[H_2CO_3]}$$

$$H_2CO_3 \propto PCO_2 \text{ because } CO_2 + H_2O \rightleftharpoons H_2CO_3$$

$$pK = 6.1$$

Generally

$$pH = pK + \log \frac{[base]}{[acid]}$$

$$H_2CO_3 \rightleftharpoons H^+ + HCO_3^- \qquad pK = 6.1$$

$$H_2PO_4^- \rightleftharpoons H^+ + HPO_4^{2-} \qquad pK = 6.8$$

$$NH_4^+ \rightleftharpoons H^+ + NH_3 \qquad pK = 9.2$$

H⁺ and pH

pH	7.6	7.5	7.4	7.3	7.2	7.1	7.0	6.9	6.8
[H⁺] nmol/L	25	32	40	50	60	80	100	125	160

The Renal System at a Glance, Fourth Edition. Chris O'Callaghan. © 2017 John Wiley & Sons, Ltd. Published 2017 by John Wiley & Sons, Ltd.
Companion website: www.ataglanceseries.com/renalsystem

Metabolic acid production and dietary H^+ intake must be balanced by acid excretion. Carbon dioxide produced by oxidative metabolism is excreted by the lungs, but other acids, such as sulfuric and phosphoric acids, are excreted by the kidneys. Protein metabolism produces 40–80 mmol of hydrogen ions per day, but normal extracellular pH is 7.35–7.45 or 35–45 nmol/L. As acid production is in the millimolar (10^{-3} mol/L) range, and yet plasma levels are regulated at the nanomolar (10^{-9} mol/L) level, buffers are needed to prevent huge swings in free hydrogen ion concentration. Buffers can bind H^+ and so protect the body from the effects of any excess H^+. Nevertheless, buffers do not alter the body's overall H^+ load, which must ultimately be excreted if the buffering capacity of the body is not to be exceeded and a dangerous pH reached.

Physiological buffers

Buffers in both blood and urine reduce the concentration of free H^+ ions. Buffers are weak acids or weak bases that are not fully dissociated. An acid can donate H^+ ions and a base can accept them. At a given H^+ concentration, a defined amount of buffer exists as acid (HA) and a defined amount as base (A^-). The ratio of buffer acid to buffer base at a given H^+ concentration is defined by the dissociation constant for an acid-base couple (pK). For a given acid-base pair, altering the ratio of the acid to the base alters the pH.

Different buffer pairs within the body are in equilibrium with each other. The main extracellular buffer is the bicarbonate system; the main intracellular buffers are sodium phosphate (Na_2HPO_4/NaH_2PO_4) and proteins. Proteins can act as acids or bases because they contain both acidic and basic amino acid side chains. As these buffer systems are all in equilibrium, altering the bicarbonate system will change body pH, which resets the ratio of acid to base in the other buffers. The lungs alter the bicarbonate system by altering the carbon dioxide partial pressure (PCO_2) and the kidneys by altering the (HCO_3^-) concentration.

Acid excretion

The body can excrete acid by the urinary loss of H^+ ions associated with a buffer or by the excretion of H^+ ions as ammonium ions (NH_4^+). As hydrogen secretion into urine is inhibited below pH 4.4, this is the minimum urine pH that can be obtained. The presence of buffers in the urine allows far greater quantities of H^+ ions to be excreted above this pH than would be possible if only free H^+ ions were excreted. This is because most of the excreted H^+ are bound by the buffers and do not have a major effect on the urine pH. The major independent urinary buffer is sodium phosphate. Phosphate that is not bound to protein is freely filtered in the glomerulus and around 75% is reabsorbed. The rest is available for buffering in the urine. Nevertheless, phosphate excretion cannot be increased indefinitely and as the pK_a of phosphate is 6.8, around 90% of its buffering capacity is used up before the urinary pH drops below 5.7. Consequently, most acid excretion occurs as a result of ammonium ion excretion.

Charge and permeability

A number of compounds such as CO_2, H_2O, and NH_3 can cross cell membranes relatively easily. However, if they are converted into their charged counterparts, such as HCO_3^-, NH_4^+, H^+, OH^-, these charged particles are much less able to diffuse across the cell membrane.

Carbonic anhydrase

Carbonic anhydrase (CA) catalyzes the reaction

$$OH^- + CO_2 \rightleftharpoons HCO_3^-$$

As water must first dissociate to form H^+ and OH^- for this reaction, it is usually written as

$$H_2O + CO_2 \rightleftharpoons H_2CO_3 \rightleftharpoons H^+ + HCO_3^-$$

The active site of the enzyme is a cone-shaped cavity with a zinc ion at its narrowest point. There are multiple isoforms of carbonic anhydrase. In the kidney, 95% of the carbonic anhydrase is carbonic anhydrase type 2, which is free in the cytosol, and 5% is membrane associated (mainly type 4 at the apical luminal membrane).

20 Renal acid-base handling

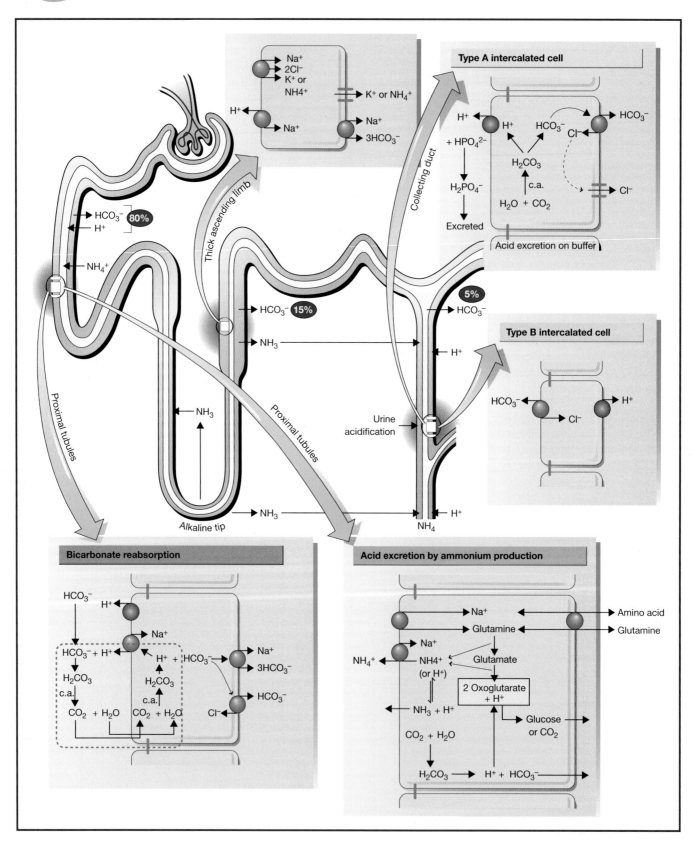

The Renal System at a Glance, Fourth Edition. Chris O'Callaghan. © 2017 John Wiley & Sons, Ltd. Published 2017 by John Wiley & Sons, Ltd.
Companion website: www.ataglanceseries.com/renalsystem

Bicarbonate reabsorption

Bicarbonate is freely filtered in the glomerulus, but most of the filtered bicarbonate is subsequently reabsorbed to maintain normal plasma bicarbonate concentration and therefore the plasma pH. Bicarbonate reabsorption depends on the secretion of H^+ ions into the lumen of the tubule. These H^+ ions are recycled by carbonic anhydrase (see Chapter 19) and there is no net acid excreted.

Hydrogen ion secretion and its effects

• When secreted H^+ ions interact with bicarbonate in the filtrate, the end result is bicarbonate reabsorption.

• When secreted H^+ ions interact with a urinary buffer (mainly phosphate or NH_3), the end result is the excretion of acid. When buffered acid excretion occurs, the new bicarbonate generated in the renal cells by carbonic anhydrase is added to the blood.

Early in the nephron, secreted H^+ ions are used to reabsorb bicarbonate. In the more distal nephron, when this bicarbonate reabsorption is complete, secreted H^+ ions interact with phosphate buffers and net acid excretion occurs. This happens because the pK_a of the bicarbonate system is 6.1, whereas that of the phosphate system is 6.8. At the initial filtrate pH of around 7.4 (similar to plasma), there is a much greater supply of bicarbonate base (HCO_3^-) than of phosphate base (HPO_4^{2-}). As bicarbonate is reabsorbed, urinary pH falls and the buffers accept H^+ ions.

Ammonia handling and acid-base balance

Tubular cells, principally those in the proximal tubule, metabolize glutamine to produce ammonia and, ultimately, glucose and bicarbonate. Glutamine can enter the cell from the tubular lumen via the B0AT1 sodium-amino acid co-transporter or from blood via the basal LAT2 amino acid exchanger. The bicarbonate enters the blood and the NH_4^+ ions (which effectively carry an H^+ ion) are excreted in the urine. NH_3 enters the filtrate from the tubular cells by simple diffusion and is protonated in the lumen to form NH_4^+, which cannot diffuse out of the tubules. The **NHE3** Na^+/H^+ exchanger can also transport NH_4^+ into the tubule. In the thick ascending limb of the loop of Henle, NH_4^+ can be transported out of the lumen in place of K^+ on the **NKCC2** co-transporter. Also, as the tip of the loop of Henle is alkaline, NH_4^+ in the filtrate dissociates to form NH_3 and this diffuses into the interstitium. Subsequently, ammonia can diffuse back from both these sites into the thin descending limb, to be recycled in a counter-current fashion. It can also diffuse into the acidified distal tubules where it is protonated to NH_4^+ and excreted in the urine.

Tubular handling of H^+ and HCO_3^-

Proximal tubule

Of the filtered bicarbonate, 80% is reabsorbed in the proximal tubule. Most proximal tubule H^+ secretion serves this purpose and does not contribute to net acid excretion. Carbonic anhydrase in the proximal tubule cell cytoplasm and the tubular lumen facilitates the reabsorption of bicarbonate by recycling the secreted H^+ ions.

Most H^+ ions enter the filtrate via the **NHE3** Na^+/H^+ exchanger at the apical membrane of the tubular cells. This protein is one of a family of molecules with 10–12 transmembrane regions, and is inhibited by cAMP and protein kinase A-mediated phosphorylation of its cytoplasmic tail. Na^+/H^+ exchange is linked to sodium reabsorption and is dependent ultimately on the activity of the basolateral Na^+/K^+ ATPase. The basolateral $Na^+/3HCO_3^-$ co-transporter (**NBC**) carries most of the bicarbonate out of the cell and into the peritubular plasma. Some sodium-dependent $3HCO_3^-/Cl^-$ counter-transport may also occur.

Loop of Henle

A further 10–15% of filtered bicarbonate is reabsorbed in the thick ascending limb of the loop of Henle. The mechanisms responsible are similar to those in the proximal tubule and again involve carbonic anhydrase.

Distal nephron

Here, secreted H^+ ions either contribute to the reabsorption of any remaining bicarbonate or interact with urinary buffers to allow acid excretion. H^+ ions are buffered by phosphate and NH_3, which diffuses in from the medullary interstitium. Secreted H^+ ions that interact with buffers are not recycled and the new bicarbonate formed in the cell enters the blood. In the early distal tubule, Na^+/H^+ exchange still mediates most H^+ secretion but, more distally, the H^+ ATPase performs this role. The connecting tubule and cortical collecting duct contain two types of intercalated cells that are rich in carbonic anhydrase.

• **Type A** intercalated cells secrete H^+ ions. Principally, this is performed by an apical **H^+ ATPase**, but also to a lesser extent by an H^+/K^+ ATPase similar to that in the stomach (see Chapter 16). The bicarbonate generated in the cell exits basolaterally via the **AE1** $3HCO_3^-/Cl^-$ anion exchanger.

• **Type B** intercalated cells are similar to functionally inverted type A cells with a basolateral H^+ ATPase and an apical AE1 HCO_3^-/Cl^- exchanger. Present only in the connecting tubule and cortical collecting duct, these cells secrete bicarbonate, but their role in normal acid-base homeostasis is unclear.

The principal cells play no direct role in acid-base handling, but their reabsorption of sodium generates a negative potential in the lumen, promoting H^+ secretion by type A intercalated cells.

21 Acid-base regulation and responses to acid-base disturbances

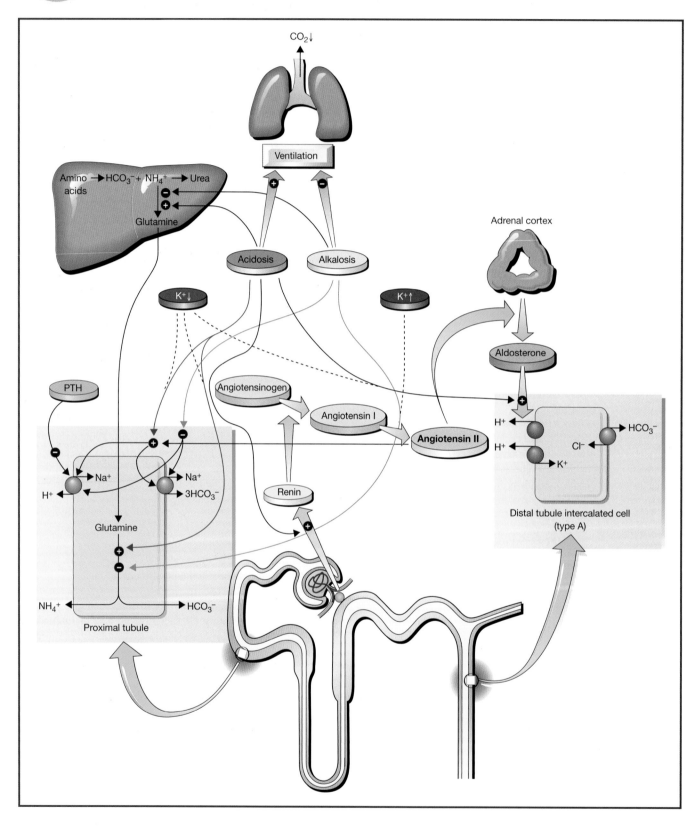

The Renal System at a Glance, Fourth Edition. Chris O'Callaghan. © 2017 John Wiley & Sons, Ltd. Published 2017 by John Wiley & Sons, Ltd.
Companion website: www.ataglanceseries.com/renalsystem

Total body pH can be regulated by controlling the ratio of CO_2 (acid) to HCO_3^- (base) in plasma.

Ventilation controls the CO_2 level and the kidney controls the HCO_3^- level. Disorders of acid-base metabolism can therefore arise either from excess acid or base, or from diseases altering CO_2 or HCO_3^- levels. In a respiratory acid-base disturbance, the primary disorder alters the CO_2 level whereas, in a metabolic acid-base disturbance, the primary disorder alters the HCO_3^- level either directly or by the addition of acid or base to the body. In a mixed disorder, there may be both respiratory and metabolic disturbances. When either HCO_3^- or CO_2 levels change, the pH can be brought back toward normal by altering the other buffer partner in the same direction (see Chapter 19).

Renal responses to acid-base abnormalities

Metabolic acidosis

With metabolic acidosis, plasma and filtrate bicarbonate concentrations are low. Acidosis directly stimulates proximal tubular glutamine metabolism, producing NH_4^+ for excretion and generating new bicarbonate. Acidosis also increases H^+ secretion and therefore bicarbonate reabsorption in both the proximal and the distal tubule. In the proximal tubule, there is increased synthesis of the apical NHE3 Na^+/H^+ exchangers and increased activity of the basolateral NBC $Na^+/3HCO_3^-$ co-transporters. In the distal tubule, there are increased numbers of H^+ ATPases in the apical membranes of type A intercalated cells. Acidosis directly stimulates renin release, which raises angiotensin II production, and aldosterone secretion, which also promotes H^+ ATPase activity in type A intercalated cells.

Metabolic alkalosis

Bicarbonate levels are high in metabolic alkalosis and this inhibits renal ammoniagenesis. The renal response to alkalosis depends on **chloride**. Low chloride levels exacerbate metabolic alkalosis. In the collecting duct, active secretion of H^+ by the H^+ ATPase is associated with passive co-transport of chloride to maintain electroneutrality. If plasma and therefore filtrate chloride levels are low, the gradient for chloride movement into the filtrate is increased. This enhances H^+ ion secretion and with it bicarbonate reabsorption. In the collecting tubule, type B intercalated cells secrete bicarbonate in exchange for chloride ions, and bicarbonate secretion is inhibited if chloride levels are low.

Respiratory acidosis and alkalosis

In **acute respiratory acidosis**, excess CO_2 shifts the carbonic anhydrase reaction toward HCO_3^- production and there is a slight increase in HCO_3^-. However, in chronic respiratory acidosis, there is enhanced bicarbonate reabsorption in the proximal and distal tubules. In the proximal tubule, there is increased apical Na^+/H^+ exchange and basolateral $Na^+/3HCO_3^-$ co-transport. In the distal tubule, there is increased apical membrane H^+ ATPase insertion and enhanced expression of the AE1 HCO_3^-/Cl^- exchanger.

In **respiratory alkalosis**, the changes are the opposite of those in respiratory acidosis, and plasma bicarbonate levels fall as a result of reduced renal bicarbonate reabsorption. Low CO_2 levels also trigger an acute mild increase in lactic and citric acid production.

Role of the liver in acid-base metabolism

The hepatic catabolism of proteins that contain sulfur and PO_4^{3-} generates acid. Most other hepatic protein catabolism is neutral and produces both HCO_3^- and NH_4^+. Most of the NH_4^+ reacts with the HCO_3^- to form urea and has no impact on acid-base balance. However, some of the NH_4^+ is diverted to hepatic glutamine synthesis. The glutamine travels in the blood to the proximal tubule for renal ammoniagenesis. Each NH_4^+ excreted in the kidney is associated with one new HCO_3^- added to the blood. Both hepatic glutamine synthesis and renal ammoniagenesis are enhanced by acidosis and reduced by alkalosis.

Role of the lungs in acid-base metabolism

As CO_2 diffuses well and is highly soluble, there is a relatively linear relationship between ventilation and plasma CO_2 levels. A fall in pH triggers arterial chemoreceptors, particularly in the carotid body, and increases the ventilation rate.

Effects of potassium on acid-base disorders

Acidosis causes H^+ ions to enter cells and potassium ions exit to maintain electroneutrality. Thus, *acidosis can cause hyperkalemia and alkalosis can cause hypokalemia*. In addition:

• hyperkalemia promotes acidosis. Potassium inhibits proximal tubule NH_4^+ production and, in the loop of Henle, K^+ competes with NH_4^+ at the NKCC2 co-transporter, impairing NH_4^+ excretion; and

• hypokalemia promotes alkalosis. Potassium depletion enhances proximal NH_4^+ production, Na^+/H^+ exchange, and the activity of the $Na^+/3HCO_3^-$ co-transport. Low intracellular potassium levels stimulate the collecting duct H^+/K^+ ATPase, promoting H^+ secretion, K^+ reabsorption, and HCO_3^- reabsorption.

Hormonal effects

Aldosterone increases acid secretion by the H^+ ATPase in type A intercalated cells in the distal tubule. **Angiotensin II** upregulates the NHE3 Na^+/H^+ exchangers and NBC $Na^+/3HCO_3^-$ co-transporter and therefore promotes H^+ secretion and bicarbonate reabsorption. **Parathyroid hormone** (PTH) stimulates proximal ammoniagenesis, and decreases proximal bicarbonate reabsorption by inhibiting Na^+/H^+ exchange. **Renal nerves** and **catecholamines** also stimulate NHE3 activity, promoting alkalosis.

22 Clinical disorders of acid-base metabolism and metabolic acidosis

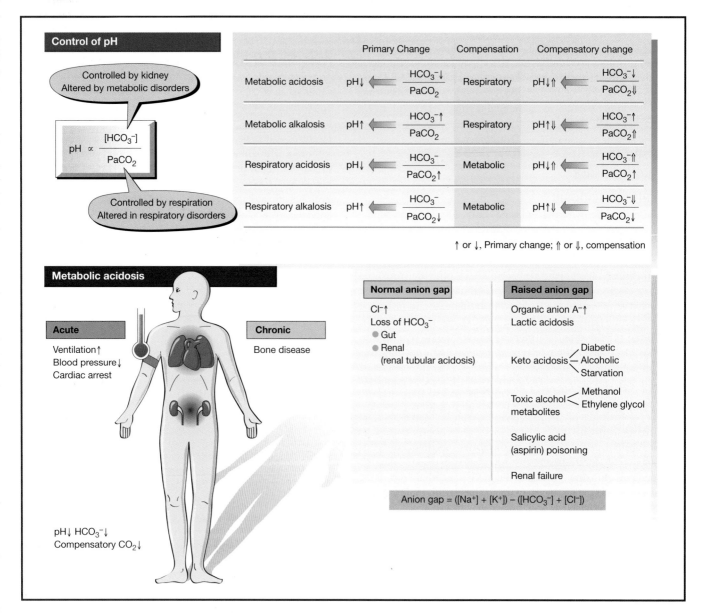

Control of pH

Controlled by kidney
Altered by metabolic disorders

$$pH \propto \frac{[HCO_3^-]}{PaCO_2}$$

Controlled by respiration
Altered in respiratory disorders

		Primary Change	Compensation	Compensatory change
Metabolic acidosis	pH↓ ←	$\frac{HCO_3^-↓}{PaCO_2}$	Respiratory	pH↓⇑ ← $\frac{HCO_3^-↓}{PaCO_2⇓}$
Metabolic alkalosis	pH↑ ←	$\frac{HCO_3^-↑}{PaCO_2}$	Respiratory	pH↑⇓ ← $\frac{HCO_3^-↑}{PaCO_2⇑}$
Respiratory acidosis	pH↓ ←	$\frac{HCO_3^-}{PaCO_2↑}$	Metabolic	pH↓⇑ ← $\frac{HCO_3^-⇑}{PaCO_2↑}$
Respiratory alkalosis	pH↑ ←	$\frac{HCO_3^-}{PaCO_2↓}$	Metabolic	pH↑⇓ ← $\frac{HCO_3^-⇓}{PaCO_2↓}$

↑ or ↓, Primary change; ⇑ or ⇓, compensation

Metabolic acidosis

Acute

Ventilation↑
Blood pressure↓
Cardiac arrest

Chronic

Bone disease

pH↓ HCO_3^-↓
Compensatory CO_2↓

Normal anion gap

Cl^-↑
Loss of HCO_3^-
● Gut
● Renal
  (renal tubular acidosis)

Raised anion gap

Organic anion A^-↑
Lactic acidosis

Keto acidosis — Diabetic
— Alcoholic
— Starvation

Toxic alcohol — Methanol
metabolites — Ethylene glycol

Salicylic acid
(aspirin) poisoning

Renal failure

Anion gap = $([Na^+] + [K^+]) - ([HCO_3^-] + [Cl^-])$

Acid-base disorders can seem confusing, but there are only a few common disorders and they are relatively easy to distinguish. It is essential to establish the nature of the disturbance before trying to determine the cause. To do this, the following questions are useful.

• Is the patient acidotic or alkalotic? This is determined by the **arterial** pH.

• Is ventilation compensating for the pH change or contributing to it? This is determined by the **arterial P**CO_2 and distinguishes metabolic from respiratory disorders, respectively.

• If there is a metabolic acidosis, is the **anion gap normal or elevated**? This determines whether acid has been acquired or bicarbonate lost.

• Last, what is the **diagnosis**?

Metabolic acidosis

Metabolic acidosis arises from the gain of acid or the loss of base as bicarbonate.

Clinical features

Acidotic patients have increased ventilation, which can be deep and rapid (Kussmaul's respiration). At low pH, the blood pressure falls as a result of reduced peripheral resistance and impaired myocardial contractility, resulting from poor actin–myosin cross-bridge cycling. Pulmonary edema and, ultimately, ventricular arrest can occur. Chronic metabolic acidosis causes hypercalciuria and buffering of acid by bone causes loss of calcium from the bone. Serum potassium is often elevated, as a result of a shift of potassium out of the cells. In pure metabolic acidosis, the pH is low, HCO_3^- is low, and PCO_2 is low to compensate.

The Renal System at a Glance, Fourth Edition. Chris O'Callaghan. © 2017 John Wiley & Sons, Ltd. Published 2017 by John Wiley & Sons, Ltd.
Companion website: www.ataglanceseries.com/renalsystem

The anion gap in metabolic acidosis

The **anion gap** is the difference between the measured cations and the measured anions in plasma. As plasma is always electrically neutral, this difference is made up by unmeasured anions. These are usually proteins, organic acids, sulfate, and phosphate, and the normal anion gap is around 6–16 mmol/L. In metabolic acidosis:

• an **increased anion gap** occurs if a new acid is added to the body. This dissociates producing free H^+ (which uses up bicarbonate) and anions (which take the place of the bicarbonate); and

• a **normal anion gap** occurs if there is simple loss of bicarbonate. This causes a compensatory rise in plasma chloride concentration, so the anion gap is normal.

$$\text{Anion gap} = ([Na^+] + [K^+]) - ([HCO_3^-] + [Cl^-])$$

Causes of normal anion gap metabolic acidosis

Gut bicarbonate loss

Bicarbonate can be lost from the gut in diarrhea, or from the small intestinal, pancreatic, or biliary drains, and from fistulae. Ileal conduits that divert urine to the bowel, especially ureterosigmoidostomies, cause acidosis because the bowel mucosa exchanges chloride in the urine for bicarbonate.

Renal bicarbonate loss

Loss of bicarbonate in the urine causes acidosis and is the basis of some renal tubular acidoses (see Chapter 24).

Increased sodium chloride intake

Excess infusion of intravenous fluid can contribute to metabolic acidosis. Plasma is normally slightly alkaline with a pH of 7.35–7.45. Water is relatively slightly acidic with a pH of 6.8–7.0 depending on the temperature. Therefore, when water without buffer is added to the plasma with sodium chloride or dextrose solutions, the acidity of the plasma will increase. This is sometimes termed "dilutional acidosis." The plasma chloride level is lower than the plasma sodium level, so administration of sodium chloride will cause a proportionately higher rise in plasma chloride than sodium.

Causes of increased anion gap metabolic acidosis

Addition of acid

Lactic acid is the end product of anaerobic metabolism and is normally metabolized to bicarbonate by the liver in an oxygen-dependent pathway. It accumulates when there is reduced oxygen delivery to the tissues, impaired oxidative metabolism, or reduced liver function. Lactic acidosis usually occurs in very sick, hemodynamically shocked, or septic patients, and indicates inadequate tissue oxygenation, often combined with impaired lactate metabolism caused by poor liver perfusion.

The ketoacids, β-hydroxybutyric acid and acetoacetic acid, accumulate during diabetic ketoacidosis and are present in blood and urine. The absence of insulin promotes their production and inhibits their catabolism. In people with noninsulin-dependent (Type 2) diabetes, the small amount of endogenous insulin present prevents these changes. Alcoholic ketoacidosis and starvation also produce excess plasma and urine ketones. Alcoholic ketoacidosis probably represents a combination of alcohol toxicity and starvation.

Toxic alcohols such as methanol and ethylene glycol (antifreeze) cause a difference between the predicted osmolality (calculated from the concentrations of ions, glucose, and urea) and the measured osmolality. In both cases, alcohol dehydrogenase metabolizes the alcohol to a more seriously toxic metabolite. This can be prevented by saturating the enzyme with ethanol, while the poisonous alcohol is removed by dialysis. Methanol typically causes abdominal pain, vomiting, headache, and visual disturbances or blindness resulting from severe retinitis. Ethylene glycol causes similar symptoms to methanol, as well as acute and chronic renal failure, but not usually retinitis.

Aspirin poisoning triggers increased ventilation, causing an early respiratory alkalosis. However, salicylic acid itself then causes a metabolic acidosis. There is often tinnitus and nausea, hyperventilation and sometimes noncardiogenic pulmonary edema, and an elevated prothrombin time. Seizures and death can occur if cerebral tissue levels are high.

Rare inborn errors of metabolism, such as the aminoacidemias, can produce metabolic acidosis presenting after birth.

Failure of acid excretion

Acute or chronic renal failure leads to the retention of phosphate, sulfate, and organic anions. Initially, there is buffering by bicarbonate and then also by bone and intracellular buffers.

Treatment of metabolic acidosis

The primary abnormality should be corrected. In principle, acute intravenous bicarbonate administration could acutely worsen intracellular acidosis by producing CO_2, which diffuses into cells and lowers the intracellular pH. In practice, this is seldom a problem and bicarbonate is often administered. Excess acid should be removed, either by further metabolism in the case of lactate and ketones, or by urinary excretion or dialysis for other acids. Slow bicarbonate administration will correct the bicarbonate deficiency in hyperchloremic metabolic acidosis. Hyperkalemia should be corrected as a raised potassium level inhibits acid excretion by interfering with NH_4^+ production (see Chapter 21).

23 Metabolic alkalosis, respiratory acidosis, and respiratory alkalosis

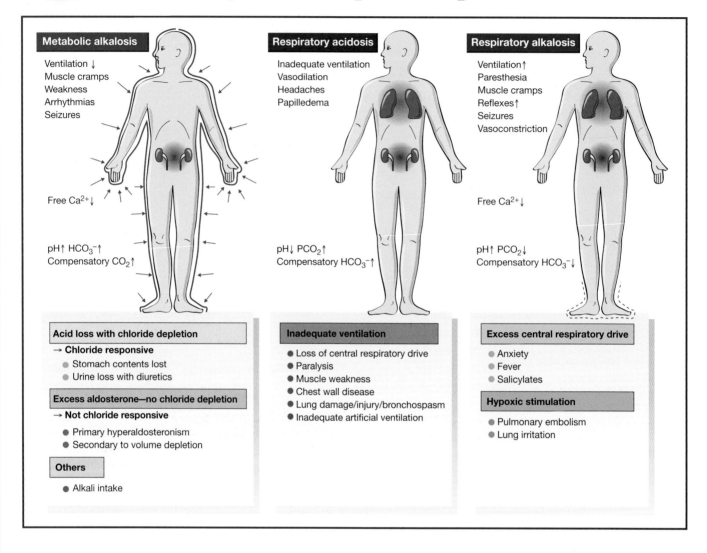

Metabolic alkalosis

Ventilation ↓
Muscle cramps
Weakness
Arrhythmias
Seizures

Free Ca^{2+}↓

pH↑ HCO_3^-↑
Compensatory CO_2↑

Respiratory acidosis

Inadequate ventilation
Vasodilation
Headaches
Papilledema

pH↓ PCO_2↑
Compensatory HCO_3^-↑

Respiratory alkalosis

Ventilation↑
Paresthesia
Muscle cramps
Reflexes↑
Seizures
Vasoconstriction

Free Ca^{2+}↓

pH↑ PCO_2↓
Compensatory HCO_3^-↓

Acid loss with chloride depletion

→ **Chloride responsive**
- Stomach contents lost
- Urine loss with diuretics

Excess aldosterone—no chloride depletion

→ **Not chloride responsive**
- Primary hyperaldosteronism
- Secondary to volume depletion

Others
- Alkali intake

Inadequate ventilation
- Loss of central respiratory drive
- Paralysis
- Muscle weakness
- Chest wall disease
- Lung damage/injury/bronchospasm
- Inadequate artificial ventilation

Excess central respiratory drive
- Anxiety
- Fever
- Salicylates

Hypoxic stimulation
- Pulmonary embolism
- Lung irritation

Metabolic alkalosis

In metabolic alkalosis, plasma pH and plasma bicarbonate levels are both raised. This can result from addition of bicarbonate to the blood or from loss of H^+ ions from the body. As plasma bicarbonate rises above a certain level, the concentration of bicarbonate in the filtrate exceeds the tubular threshold for bicarbonate reabsorption and the excess bicarbonate is excreted. For this reason, a severe metabolic alkalosis can arise only when the kidneys cannot excrete this excess bicarbonate. This can happen if there is inadequate renal perfusion or excess aldosterone. **Aldosterone** enhances distal bicarbonate

reabsorption in type A intercalated cells by stimulating the H^+ ATPase. Aldosterone also promotes sodium reabsorption in the distal tubule, which increases potassium loss. The hypokalemia further enhances bicarbonate reabsorption (see Chapter 21).

Factors that worsen metabolic alkalosis

Low plasma chloride

Chloride is necessary for bicarbonate excretion, and if plasma chloride concentration is low, chloride replacement is necessary to achieve efficient bicarbonate excretion. Chloride is exchanged

The Renal System at a Glance, Fourth Edition. Chris O'Callaghan. © 2017 John Wiley & Sons, Ltd. Published 2017 by John Wiley & Sons, Ltd.
Companion website: www.ataglanceseries.com/renalsystem

for bicarbonate across tubular cell membranes by the AE1 anion exchange proteins at a number of sites in the nephron. Aldosterone excess is not associated with a low chloride concentration and chloride replacement is of no benefit.

Hypovolemia

This exacerbates metabolic alkalosis by stimulating aldosterone release which increases bicarbonate reabsorption as discussed above.

Causes of metabolic alkalosis

Loss of acid from the gut or kidney

Gastric contents are acidic because the luminal, omeprazole-inhibited H^+ ATPase in parietal cells secretes acid into the stomach. Loss of gastric contents, particularly when there is repeated vomiting, as in pyloric stenosis, can cause metabolic alkalosis. There is often also volume depletion and chloride loss.

Addition of bicarbonate to the body

This can result from the ingestion or administration of bicarbonate or substances such as lactate, citrate, or acetate, which are metabolized to generate bicarbonate.

Renal dysfunction and aldosterone

Any cause of a high aldosterone level can cause a metabolic alkalosis by increasing H^+ ATPase activity and therefore bicarbonate reabsorption in the distal tubule.

Other causes

Diuretics can contribute to alkalosis by causing hypovolemia with secondary hyperaldosteronism, hypokalemia, and chloride depletion. Glycyrrhizinic acid in black licorice causes a hypokalemic metabolic alkalosis and hypertension by upregulating renal mineralocorticoid receptors, thereby enhancing the effect of aldosterone. Severe potassium depletion can cause metabolic alkalosis by its effect on the kidney. Albumin is a weak acid and so low albumin levels can contribute to metabolic alkalosis. Rare causes of metabolic alkalosis include excess citrate administration in blood products, and milk–alkali syndrome (see Chapter 27).

Clinical features

These are not specific but can include muscle cramps, weakness, dysrhythmias, and seizures. These features may relate to a reduction in free calcium that can occur when calcium ions bind to the negative charges on proteins at sites normally occupied by H^+. The normal respiratory response to metabolic alkalosis is diminished breathing, but obviously the hypoxic drive to breathing ensures that breathing maintains adequate oxygenation. There is usually hypokalemia as a result of the shift of potassium into cells.

If the underlying cause is not clinically obvious, vomiting, diuretic overuse, and primary hyperaldosteronism should be considered. Vomiting and diuretics lead to volume contraction, whereas excess mineralocorticoid leads to volume expansion.

Treatment

The underlying cause should be treated. Chloride-responsive alkalosis responds to chloride and volume replacement and improved renal hemodynamics. The increase in chloride delivery promotes distal bicarbonate secretion. Hypokalemia should be corrected. In nonchloride-responsive alkalosis, it may be necessary to block the effect of aldosterone, for example, with spironolactone or amiloride. The pH can be corrected rapidly by ventilation using inspired CO_2 and supplemental oxygen to prevent hypoxia.

Respiratory acidosis

This results from a primary decrease in ventilation as a result of depression of the respiratory center, a physical impediment to breathing, such as neurological or muscular disease, or lung injury.

An acute rise in plasma CO_2 is usually associated with a fall in oxygen levels, dyspnea, reduced consciousness, and eventually, coma. Carbon dioxide causes vasodilation, which may increase cerebral blood flow, causing headaches and raised intracranial pressure. Systemic vasodilation reduces blood pressure, and large rises in plasma CO_2 levels reduce cardiac contractility. In chronic respiratory acidosis, papilledema can occur and there may be reduced bone mineralization as a result of buffering.

Treatment must improve gas exchange. This can be done by treating any underlying disease and by artificial ventilation, or by giving doxapram hydrochloride which triggers central and peripheral chemoreceptors to stimulate ventilation.

Respiratory alkalosis

A primary increase in ventilation can occur as a result of excessive artificial ventilation or in hypoxemia, fever, brain disease, acute cardiopulmonary syndromes, septicemia, liver failure, or pregnancy, and as a side effect of drugs such as salicylates. Plasma bicarbonate falls as a result of reduced bicarbonate reabsorption in the kidney, and buffering often includes increased lactate production.

Clinically, there is neuromuscular irritability, with perioral and extremity paresthesia, muscle cramps and tinnitus, hyperreflexia, tetany, and seizures. Cerebral vasoconstriction with reduced blood flow and cardiac dysrhythmias can occur.

Treatment involves correction of the underlying disorder or inhalation of extra CO_2.

Panic attacks with hyperventilation cause transient respiratory alkalosis and are dominated by symptoms of acute hypocalcemia. The alkalosis exposes negative charges on plasma proteins that were previously bound to H^+, and the free calcium level falls as calcium ions bind to these sites. Common symptoms are paresthesia and circumoral numbness. Acute treatment can involve relaxation methods and rebreathing into a paper bag to increase carbon dioxide levels.

24 Renal tubular acidosis

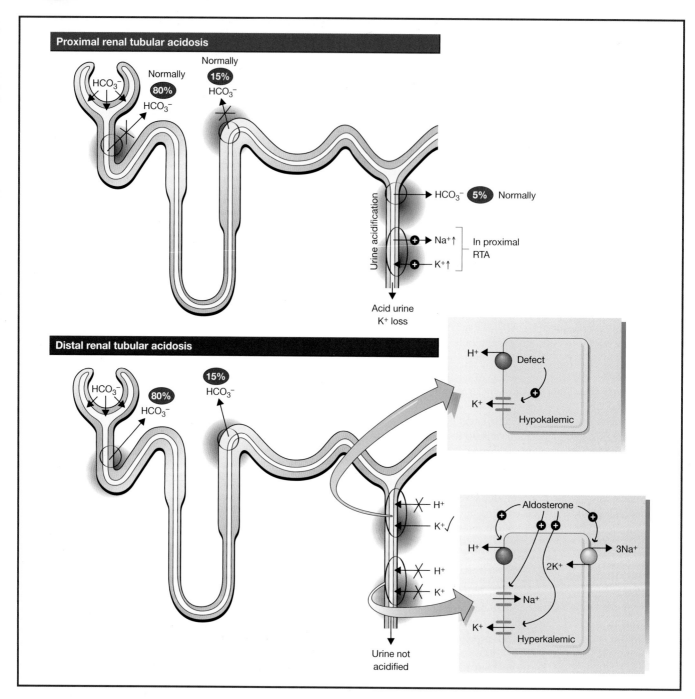

Proximal renal tubular acidosis

Normally 80%
HCO$_3^-$
HCO$_3^-$

Normally 15%
HCO$_3^-$

HCO$_3^-$ 5% Normally

Urine acidification

Na$^+$↑
K$^+$↑
} In proximal RTA

Acid urine
K$^+$ loss

Distal renal tubular acidosis

Normally 80%
HCO$_3^-$
HCO$_3^-$

15%
HCO$_3^-$

H$^+$
K$^+$✓

H$^+$
K$^+$

Urine not acidified

H$^+$
Defect
K$^+$
Hypokalemic

Aldosterone
H$^+$ 3Na$^+$
2K$^+$
Na$^+$
K$^+$
Hyperkalemic

The Renal System at a Glance, Fourth Edition. Chris O'Callaghan. © 2017 John Wiley & Sons, Ltd. Published 2017 by John Wiley & Sons, Ltd.
Companion website: www.ataglanceseries.com/renalsystem

Renal tubular acidosis occurs because the kidney is unable to excrete acid, and hyperchloremic, metabolic acidosis with a normal anion gap occurs (see Chapter 22). Proximal renal tubular acidosis is relatively rare and arises from a defect in proximal tubule bicarbonate reabsorption. It is often associated with other disorders of proximal tubule function. Distal renal tubular acidosis is more common. It produces a more severe acidosis and is associated with many systemic disorders.

Proximal renal tubular acidosis (type 2)

Proximal renal tubular acidosis occurs when proximal hydrogen ion secretion and bicarbonate reabsorption fail. In most cases, the specific molecular defects have not been identified, but there is often decreased activity of the NHE3 Na^+/H^+ exchanger and of the basolateral NBC $Na^+/3HCO_3^-$ co-transporter.

Defects in other proximal tubule functions, such as glucose, phosphate, or urate reabsorption, may be present and if so, this generalized proximal tubular dysfunction is termed Fanconi's syndrome (see Chapter 30). A defect in proximal tubule sodium handling may be responsible because most proximal tubular reabsorption relies to some extent on sodium transport. Causes include generalized damage to the proximal tubule in the context of genetic diseases such as cystinosis or by nephrotoxins such as myeloma light chains.

When proximal bicarbonate reabsorption fails, large amounts of bicarbonate reach the distal tubule. As the capacity of the distal tubule for bicarbonate reabsorption is limited, there is massive bicarbonate loss in the urine, causing acidosis. As a result, the plasma bicarbonate concentration falls and so the concentration of bicarbonate in the filtrate also falls. Eventually, the filtrate bicarbonate level falls low enough for it all to be reabsorbed in the distal tubules. At this stage, an acid urine can be excreted and the new low plasma bicarbonate level can be maintained. As a result, a severe acidosis does not occur.

Hypokalemia usually occurs because bicarbonate that is lost takes sodium and water with it. This sodium and water loss can cause volume depletion and triggers aldosterone release. Aldosterone promotes sodium reabsorption in the distal tubule in exchange for potassium. There is often osteomalacia and raised urinary calcium excretion, but urinary citrate levels are high and so stone formation is uncommon.

The diagnosis can be made by showing that the fractional excretion of an administered bicarbonate load is abnormally high when the plasma HCO_3^- level is above 20 mmol/L.

Treatment is with sodium bicarbonate and potassium supplements or potassium-sparing diuretics. Vitamin D and phosphate supplements may be required.

Distal renal tubular acidosis (type 1)

In distal renal tubular acidosis, H^+ secretion is impaired in the distal tubule and collecting ducts. In the normal distal tubule, urine is made acid and a high H^+ gradient develops. With distal renal tubular acidosis, an acidic urine cannot be produced and a severe metabolic acidosis arises. Typically, the severe acidosis mobilizes bone calcium and causes osteomalacia, nephrocalcinosis, and urinary stone formation. The molecular causes of a number of different types of distal tubular acidosis have been established. The diagnosis can be made by a failure to produce an acid urine even in response to an acid load with NH_4Cl. Distal renal tubular acidosis can be divided according to whether or not there is hyperkalemia.

Hypokalemic distal renal tubular acidosis

In these conditions, potassium handling itself is normal, but potassium is secreted instead of H^+ during sodium reabsorption, causing hypokalemia.

Secretory defects directly reduce H^+ secretion. This arises with mutation or loss of function of the H^+ ATPase and less commonly with mutations in the AE1 anion exchanger or the cellular carbonic anhydrase type II. Sjögren's syndrome causes an acquired deficiency of the H^+ ATPase.

Permeability defects caused by toxins such as amphotericin increase the permeability of the distal tubule to H^+, thus preventing an H^+ gradient from developing.

Hyperkalemic distal renal tubular acidosis

In these conditions, there is abnormally reduced potassium and H^+ secretion in the distal tubule. Hyperkalemia worsens the acidosis. This type of renal tubular acidosis is sometimes termed **type 4 renal tubular acidosis.**

Voltage defects. If distal tubule sodium reabsorption is defective, this reduces the negative luminal charge that promotes both H^+ and K^+ secretion. This can happen with generalized distal tubular damage, including that caused by urinary tract obstruction, interstitial nephritis associated with systemic lupus erythematosus, or amiloride and lithium use.

Hypoaldosteronism. In the distal tubule, aldosterone stimulates sodium reabsorption, potassium secretion, and acid secretion by the H^+ ATPase. Without aldosterone, there is sodium wasting, hyperkalemia, and acidosis. Low aldosterone levels can result from adrenal failure, inadequate renin secretion, or drugs inhibiting the renin–angiotensin II–aldosterone axis. The most common form is in diabetic nephropathy or tubulointerstitial disease, where there is deficient renin production. Ciclosporin A toxicity can have a similar effect.

Treatment of distal renal tubular acidosis involves sodium bicarbonate or sodium citrate administration. Hypokalemia should be corrected with potassium replacement and hyperkalemia can be treated with diuretics. Mineralocorticoid (aldosterone) should be replaced if deficient.

Defective ammoniagenesis

A renal tubular acidosis can arise from inadequate renal ammoniagenesis. Bicarbonate is still secreted and an acid urine is produced, but the amount of acid excreted is reduced because the buffering of NH_4^+ is unavailable. The principal causes are hyperkalemia, glucocorticoid deficiency, and loss of renal mass. Hyperkalemia suppresses ammoniagenesis, probably by displacing H^+ out of the cells. This causes intracellular alkalosis, which opposes cellular loss of the HCO_3^- produced by the ammoniagenesis. Glucocorticoid deficiency suppresses ammoniagenesis because glutamine synthesis, like skeletal muscle protein catabolism, is dependent on glucocorticoids.

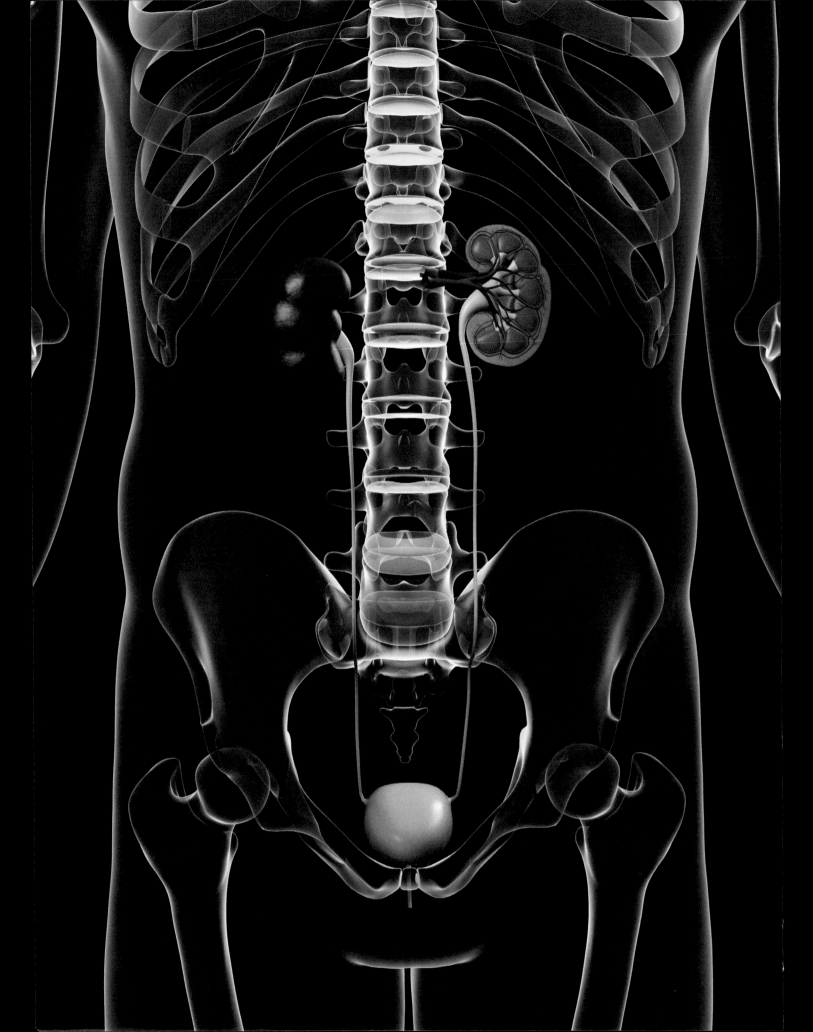

Divalent ions – calcium, phosphate and magnesium

Part 6

Chapters

25 Calcium, phosphate, and magnesium metabolism 60
26 Regulation of divalent ions and disorders of phosphate and magnesium 62
27 Hypocalcemia and hypercalcemia 64

Don't forget to visit the companion website for this book
www.ataglanceseries.com/renalsystem

25 Calcium, phosphate, and magnesium metabolism

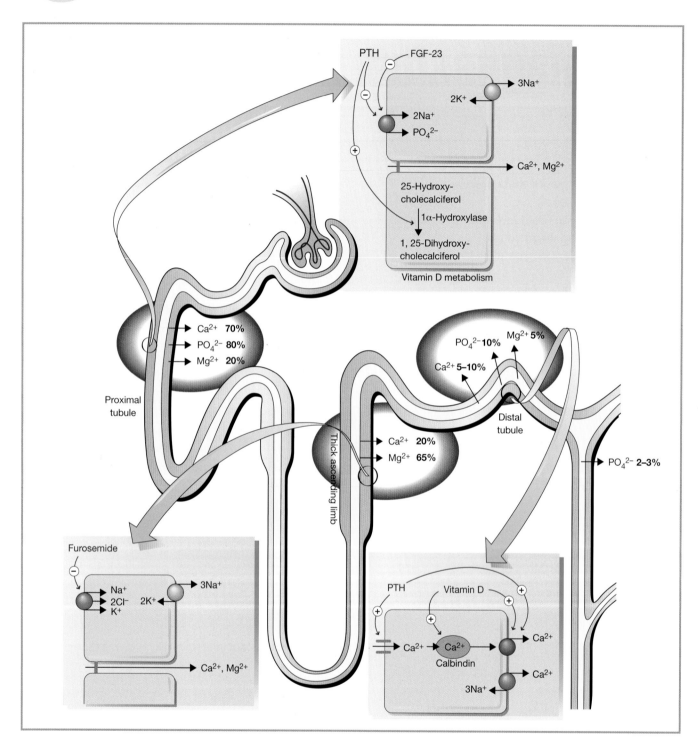

Calcium is the most prevalent divalent cation in the body, followed by magnesium; phosphate is the major divalent anion. All three occur mainly in bone. Most bone is being continuously resorbed and rebuilt at a slow rate. A more rapid bone surface exchange of calcium, phosphate and, to a lesser extent, magnesium, maintains plasma levels of these ions. Plasma calcium and phosphate concentrations are close to the saturation product (calcium ion concentration times the phosphate ion concentration or $[Ca^{2+}] \times [PO_4^{2-}]$) at which calcium phosphate complexes precipitate out of solution onto the bone matrix. Plasma values of the two ions are therefore inversely related because a rise in $[Ca^{2+}]$ or $[PO_4^{2-}]$ causes some precipitation of calcium phosphate into bone with a fall in $[PO_4^{2-}]$ or $[Ca^{2+}]$, respectively.

Inside cells, calcium regulates many processes. Intracellular calcium ion concentrations are kept very low; most calcium is bound to proteins or sequestered in the endoplasmic reticulum and mitochondria.

In plasma, calcium, phosphate, and magnesium can bind to proteins, complex with other ions (forming calcium phosphate or magnesium phosphate), or exist as free ions. Only protein-bound ions are not filtered in the glomerulus.

Calcium levels are mainly regulated by bone turnover and gut absorption, magnesium levels are regulated by renal handling, and phosphate levels by all three mechanisms.

Calcium

Of dietary calcium, 25–30% is absorbed by the gut, mainly in the duodenum and proximal jejunum. Absorption occurs by a transcellular process involving intracellular calcium-binding proteins called calbindins. Gut absorption is increased by vitamin D and during pregnancy. Total plasma calcium concentration is around 2.5 mmol/L, of which 45% is protein bound, 5% is complexed to other ions, and 50% (1.25 mmol/L) is free ionized Ca^{2+}.

Renal handling of calcium

In the glomerulus, calcium that is not protein bound is freely filtered and there is reabsorption along the nephron.

Of filtered calcium, 70% is reabsorbed in the proximal tubule and a further 20% in the thick ascending limb of the loop of Henle. This reabsorption is mainly passive and paracellular, and driven by sodium reabsorption. Sodium reabsorption causes water reabsorption, which raises tubular calcium concentration, causing calcium to diffuse out of the tubules. The positive lumen potential also encourages calcium to leave the tubule. The thin segments of the loop of Henle are impermeable to calcium.

A further 5–10% of filtered calcium is reabsorbed in the distal tubules, and there is only minor reabsorption in the collecting ducts. Calcium reabsorption in the distal tubules is active and transcellular, and is the major target for hormonal control. As the intracellular calcium concentration must be kept low, transcellular calcium movement occurs via calcium-binding proteins, as in the gut. Calcium enters the cells through the **TRPV5** epithelial Ca^{2+} channels that are activated by parathyroid hormone (PTH). It is transported across the cell by calcium-binding proteins, including the calbindins and parvalbumin. The expression of these proteins is upregulated by vitamin D. At the basolateral surface, calcium is transported out of the cell by the plasma membrane Ca^{2+} ATPase (**PMCA**) and by a $3Na^+/Ca^{2+}$ exchanger (**NCX**). The Ca^{2+} ATPase is regulated by vitamin D and PTH. If the urine becomes very acidic, this reduces the expression of the TRPV5 channels and so increases urine calcium loss.

Phosphate

About 65% of dietary phosphate is absorbed, mainly in the duodenum and jejunum by a transcellular process which is enhanced by vitamin D. Of plasma phosphate, 55% exists as free phosphate in the forms HPO_4^{2-} and $H_2PO_4^-$. These ions form a buffer pair (see Chapters 19 and 20).

Renal phosphate handling

In the glomerulus, all phosphate that is not protein bound is freely filtered and there is reabsorption along the nephron. The maximum rate of reabsorption is limited and excess filtered phosphate above a threshold level (the Tm_{Pi}) is excreted. Of filtered phosphate, 80% is reabsorbed in the proximal tubules by a transcellular process that relies on sodium reabsorption. Apical phosphate entry is by co-transport with sodium via the sodium phosphate co-transporter (**NPT2**). This transporter is downregulated by PTH. How phosphate gets out of the cell is unclear.

There is no significant phosphate transport in the loop of Henle, but the distal tubules reabsorb a further 10% of the filtered phosphate and the collecting ducts a further 2–3%. The mechanism of distal phosphate reabsorption appears to be similar to that in the proximal tubules.

Magnesium

Of the body magnesium, 54% is in bone, 45% in soft tissues, and just 1% in the extracellular fluid. In the glomerulus, magnesium that is not protein bound is freely filtered and there is reabsorption along the nephron. Only 30% is reabsorbed in the proximal tubule. The majority, 65%, is reabsorbed in the thick ascending limb by passive paracellular movement driven by the transepithelial potential. A further 5% is reabsorbed in the distal tubules. Active magnesium reabsorption occurs in the distal tubules where there are basolateral Mg^{2+} ATPases and an apical magnesium channel **TRPM6**. The permeability of TRPM6 is regulated by intracellular magnesium levels. Mutations in TRPM6 cause hypomagnesemia. Epidermal growth factor (EGF) stimulates TRPM6 and so magnesium reabsorption.

Factors influencing magnesium secretion

PTH and calcitonin increase paracellular magnesium reabsorption, possibly by influencing the permeability of the epithelial tight junctions. Both loop diuretics and thiazides increase magnesium excretion. Magnesium handling in the distal tubule and loop of Henle is directly influenced by the action of plasma magnesium ions on the Ca^{2+}/Mg^{2+} sensing receptor (**CaR**) on the capillary side of the tubular cells.

Drug effects on calcium excretion

Passive proximal calcium reabsorption depends on sodium reabsorption, so diuretics such as furosemide, which inhibit proximal or thick ascending loop sodium reabsorption, inhibit calcium reabsorption. In contrast, thiazides, which inhibit distal sodium reabsorption, do not inhibit active transcellular distal calcium reabsorption and can even enhance calcium reabsorption.

26 Regulation of divalent ions and disorders of phosphate and magnesium

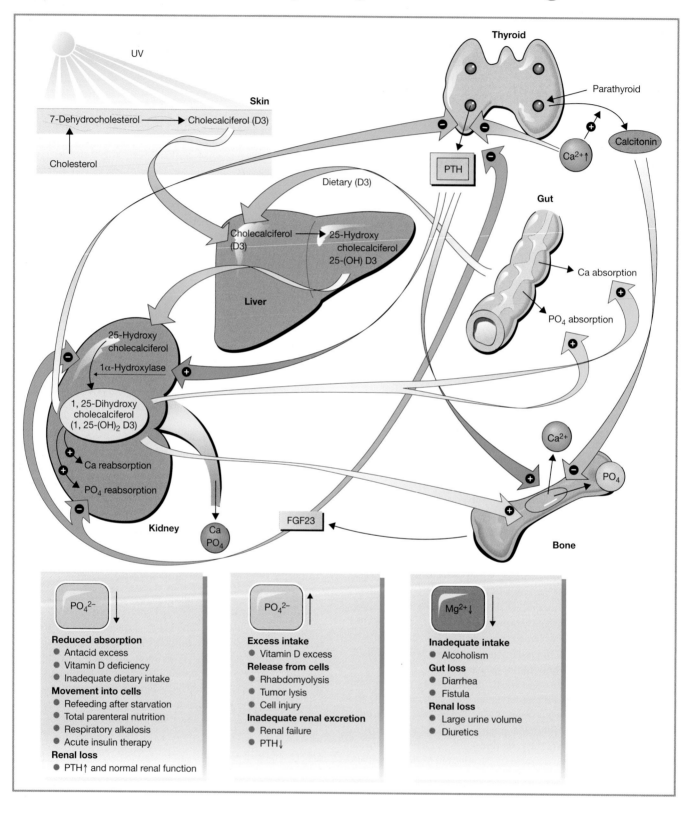

Skin

UV

7-Dehydrocholesterol ⟶ Cholecalciferol (D3)

Cholesterol

Thyroid

Parathyroid

Calcitonin

Ca²⁺↑

PTH

Dietary (D3)

Liver

Cholecalciferol (D3) ⟶ 25-Hydroxy cholecalciferol 25-(OH) D3

Gut

Ca absorption

PO₄ absorption

25-Hydroxy cholecalciferol

1α-Hydroxylase

1, 25-Dihydroxy cholecalciferol (1, 25-(OH)₂ D3)

Ca reabsorption

PO₄ reabsorption

Kidney

Ca PO₄

FGF23

Ca²⁺

PO₄

Bone

PO_4^{2-} ↓

Reduced absorption
- Antacid excess
- Vitamin D deficiency
- Inadequate dietary intake

Movement into cells
- Refeeding after starvation
- Total parenteral nutrition
- Respiratory alkalosis
- Acute insulin therapy

Renal loss
- PTH↑ and normal renal function

PO_4^{2-} ↑

Excess intake
- Vitamin D excess

Release from cells
- Rhabdomyolysis
- Tumor lysis
- Cell injury

Inadequate renal excretion
- Renal failure
- PTH↓

Mg^{2+} ↓

Inadequate intake
- Alcoholism

Gut loss
- Diarrhea
- Fistula

Renal loss
- Large urine volume
- Diuretics

The Renal System at a Glance, Fourth Edition. Chris O'Callaghan. © 2017 John Wiley & Sons, Ltd. Published 2017 by John Wiley & Sons, Ltd.
Companion website: www.ataglanceseries.com/renalsystem

Control of calcium and phosphate

Parathyroid hormone

Parathyroid hormone (PTH) is a protein secreted by the chief cells of the parathyroid gland, when extracellular ionized calcium levels fall. A G protein-coupled calcium sensing receptor (**CaR**) on the surface of chief cells influences PTH release and is itself upregulated by vitamin D. A raised calcium level normally inhibits PTH secretion. PTH receptors in the bone and kidneys act via G proteins to activate adenylyl cyclase and raise cAMP levels. Excess PTH increases serum calcium and reduces serum phosphate.

- **In bone**, PTH stimulates bone-building osteoblasts, which themselves stimulate bone-resorbing osteoclasts. There is net bone resorption with calcium and phosphate release.
- **In the kidney**, PTH has three effects: (i) it increases vitamin D synthesis; (ii) it reduces proximal tubular phosphate reabsorption which increases phosphate excretion; and (iii) it increases distal tubular calcium reabsorption by activating calcium channels.

Vitamin D

Dietary cholecalciferol is absorbed in the small intestine or synthesized in the skin by the action of ultraviolet light. The liver converts cholecalciferol to 25-hydroxycholecalciferol. This is converted by 1α-hydroxylase in the cells of the renal proximal tubule to 1,25-dihydroxycholecalciferol, the principal active form of vitamin D. Vitamin D acts on receptors in the gut, bone, and kidney to raise levels of both calcium and phosphate. The major effect is in the gut, where calcium and phosphate absorption are increased. Vitamin D enhances the action of PTH, promoting net bone resorption with calcium and phosphate release. Vitamin D stimulates renal calcium and phosphate reabsorption. The vitamin D receptor acts as a transcription factor, increasing levels of calbindins in the distal tubule cells. Vitamin D also inhibits PTH secretion from the parathyroid glands.

FGF23, calcitonin, and other hormones

The phosphatonin peptide hormone FGF23 is made by osteocytes in bone and promotes renal phosphate excretion by inhibiting phosphate reabsorption by the NPT2 sodium phosphate transporter in the proximal tubule (see Chapter 25). FGF23 also inhibits the activity of the renal 1α-hydroxylase enzyme and so reduces vitamin D synthesis in the kidney and directly inhibits PTH secretion from the parathyroid glands. The Klotho protein is expressed mainly in distal tubules and forms part of the receptor for FGF23 along with FGFR proteins. Calcitonin is a peptide secreted by thyroid C cells when plasma ionized calcium levels fall. It reduces osteoclast activity, but its role is unclear. Growth hormone (acting via insulin-like growth factor 1), insulin, and thyroxine promote renal phosphate reabsorption, whereas corticosteroids and chronic acidosis inhibit phosphate reabsorption.

Acid-base status

Acidosis increases renal phosphate excretion and alkalosis reduces renal phosphate excretion.

Hypophosphatemia

Severe hypophosphatemia indicates phosphate deficiency, but moderate hypophosphatemia is often the result of movement of phosphate into cells. Movement into cells occurs if intracellular phosphate is used up to generate phosphorylated metabolic products, such as glucose 6-phosphate and ATP. Plasma phosphate can fall if glycolysis increases suddenly, as with refeeding after starvation, starting total parenteral nutrition, giving insulin in diabetic ketoacidosis, or with respiratory alkalosis. Hypophosphatemia occurs with alcohol-related malnutrition and with ingestion of phosphate-binding antacids. PTH promotes phosphaturia, so hyperparathyroidism of any type can cause hypophosphatemia if renal function is not impaired. Vitamin D deficiency impairs calcium and phosphate absorption in the gut, lowering plasma levels of both calcium and phosphate. Severe phosphate deficiency lowers cellular ATP levels, which can impair cellular function. Hypophosphatemic rickets can be caused by mutations in the osteocyte proteins PHEX or DMP1 which normally lower FGF23 levels. These mutations cause high FGF23 levels with high urine phosphate excretion, osteomalacia and rickets.

Clinical features include weakness of skeletal, cardiac, and smooth muscle, causing dysphagia, ileus, inadequate respiratory muscle strength, and impaired myocardial contractility. Neurological problems include paresthesia, confusion, seizures, and coma. Treatment is with oral sodium phosphate or potassium phosphate. Intravenous phosphate replacement can cause severe hypocalcemia and is used only with severe phosphate depletion.

Hyperphosphatemia

Hyperphosphatemia can result from reduced urinary phosphate excretion, excessive phosphate intake, or phosphate release from cells. Renal failure is the commonest cause of severe hyperphosphatemia. As PTH promotes phosphate excretion, hypoparathyroidism can cause hyperphosphatemia. Excess vitamin D promotes excess phosphate absorption in the gut and hyperphosphatemia. Chemotherapy, tumor lysis, and rhabdomyolysis all release phosphate from cells.

Clinical features include those of hypocalcemia if it is present, such as tetany. If phosphate is elevated and calcium is not low, soft tissue calcification can occur. Treatment is by hydration with saline, which promotes phosphaturia if renal function is normal (for treatment in renal failure see Chapter 44).

Hypomagnesemia and hypermagnesemia

Magnesium is required by many essential enzymes and stabilizes excitable cell membranes, including those in the heart. Intracellular magnesium can regulate both K^+ and Ca^{2+} channels, and promotes intracellular potassium retention by stimulating the Na^+/K^+ ATPase.

Hypomagnesemia is usually caused by magnesium loss from the gut or kidneys or inadequate intake, especially in people with alcohol problems. Clinically, symptoms are neurological and muscular, resembling those of hypocalcemia. There may be tetany, Chvostek's sign, and Trousseau's sign (see Chapter 27), seizures, and cardiac dysrhythmias, especially ventricular dysrhythmias. ECG changes include a prolonged P–R interval, QRS widening, T-wave inversion, and prominent U waves. Hypomagnesemia can cause hypokalemia (see Chapter 18). Treatment is with oral or intravenous magnesium chloride.

Hypermagnesemia is rare and is usually the result of excess magnesium intake or administration. Clinical features include bradycardia, hypotension, reduced consciousness, and respiratory depression. Treatment involves removal of excess magnesium, using furosemide and hydration or dialysis. Calcium administration reverses some of the dangerous effects of magnesium on the heart.

27 Hypocalcemia and hypercalcemia

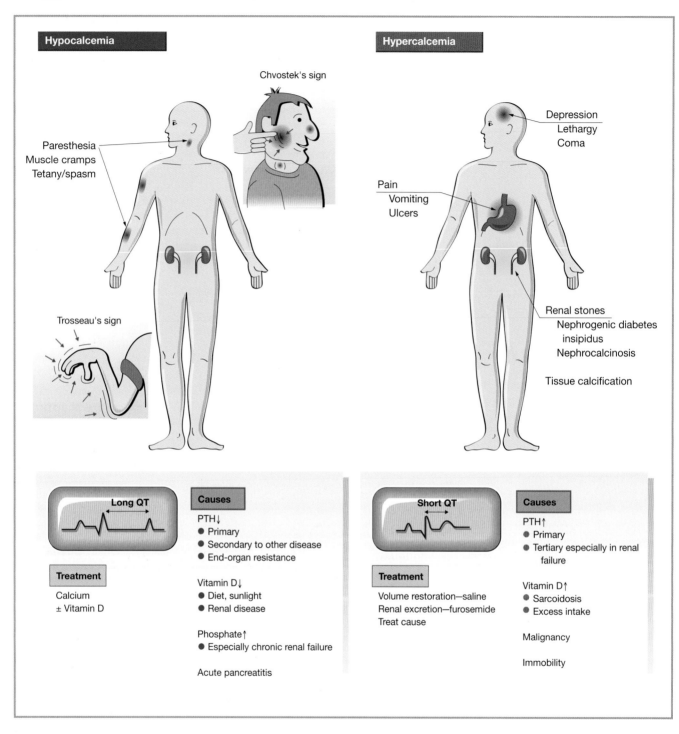

Hypocalcemia

Chvostek's sign

Paresthesia
Muscle cramps
Tetany/spasm

Trosseau's sign

Long QT

Treatment
Calcium
± Vitamin D

Causes
PTH↓
● Primary
● Secondary to other disease
● End-organ resistance

Vitamin D↓
● Diet, sunlight
● Renal disease

Phosphate↑
● Especially chronic renal failure

Acute pancreatitis

Hypercalcemia

Depression
Lethargy
Coma

Pain
Vomiting
Ulcers

Renal stones
Nephrogenic diabetes
insipidus
Nephrocalcinosis

Tissue calcification

Short QT

Treatment
Volume restoration—saline
Renal excretion—furosemide
Treat cause

Causes
PTH↑
● Primary
● Tertiary especially in renal
failure

Vitamin D↑
● Sarcoidosis
● Excess intake

Malignancy

Immobility

Around 40% of serum calcium is protein bound, but it is the concentration of free calcium ions that is biologically relevant. Changes in protein concentration alter the total calcium concentration, but the free calcium ion concentration usually remains normal. An increase in H^+ or a very large increase in Na^+ can displace Ca^{2+} ions from their binding sites on proteins. There are algorithms to estimate these effects but, if there is doubt, the free Ca^{2+} should be measured directly.

Hypocalcemia

Causes

Vitamin D deficiency

Vitamin D deficiency can result from inadequate nutrition, inadequate sun exposure, or renal damage. It causes hypocalcemia and hypophosphatemia. Vitamin D is fat soluble, and fat malabsorption as a result of pancreatic, biliary, or small intestinal disease can cause vitamin D deficiency. Vitamin D-dependent rickets is an autosomal recessive disorder caused by a deficiency of renal 1α-hydroxylase.

Hypoparathyroidism

Primary hypoparathyroidism can be sporadic and idiopathic. Familial forms result from mutations in the parathyroid hormone (PTH) gene or the DiGeorge syndrome of underdeveloped parathyroid and thymic tissues. Secondary hypoparathyroidism describes parathyroid damage that is secondary to another disease process, such as iron deposition in thalassemia, copper deposition in Wilson's disease, or autoimmune diseases involving several endocrine organs (especially the adrenals). Pseudohypoparathyroidism is a rare genetic defect. Cells do not respond to PTH because of deficiency in a G protein, which stimulates adenyl cyclase. Clinical features include hypocalcemia, hyperphosphatemia, learning disorders, short stature, and abnormally short metacarpal and metatarsal bones. Pseudo-pseudohypoparathyroidism has the same phenotype but no biochemical abnormalities.

Hyperphosphatemia and other causes

Hyperphosphatemia causes hypocalcemia by forming calcium phosphate complexes, which are deposited in bone or other tissues. Acute pancreatitis lowers serum calcium, probably because calcium forms soap-like precipitates with lipid derivatives in the peritoneum. Rarely, bone-forming malignancies such as prostatic and breast cancer can sequester calcium in bone.

Clinical features

There is neuromuscular irritability with paresthesia, circumoral numbness, muscle cramps, tetany, laryngospasm, and sometimes seizures or psychosis. Chvostek's and Trousseau's signs may be present. *Chvostek's sign* is a facial muscle twitch when the facial nerve is tapped below the zygomatic bone. *Trousseau's sign* is spasm with hyperextended fingers and metacarpophalangeal flexion, when a sphygmomanometer cuff is inflated for 3 min around the upper arm. Cardiac abnormalities include a *prolonged Q–T interval*, peaked T waves, and rarely ventricular fibrillation or heart block.

Treatment

Treat symptomatic acute hypocalcemia with intravenous calcium gluconate or calcium chloride. Chronic hypocalcemia is treated with oral calcium replacement, often with vitamin D. Magnesium levels must be corrected if low. Thiazides can raise calcium levels. High phosphate levels should be lowered to avoid calcium phosphate deposition in tissues when calcium is given.

Hypercalcemia
Causes

Hyperparathyroidism

Primary hyperparathyroidism is the most common cause of hypercalcemia, especially in elderly women. The usual cause is primary hyperplasia or a single parathyroid adenoma. Adenomas can be familial. Adenomas can be associated with other endocrine abnormalities, including the multiple endocrine neoplasia (MEN) syndromes. Treatment involves surgical removal of parathyroid

tissue. In **secondary hyperparathyroidism**, the calcium level is low and excess PTH is the appropriate response to correct the low calcium. **Tertiary hyperparathyroidism** arises following long-standing secondary hyperparathyroidism, when the parathyroid glands continue to secrete excess PTH autonomously, even when calcium levels have risen. The continued PTH secretion causes a high calcium level as in primary hyperparathyroidism.

Malignancy

This is the second commonest cause of hypercalcemia. Typical causes are squamous cell lung carcinoma, metastatic breast carcinoma, or kidney, ovary, and hematological malignancies (especially myeloma). Hypercalcemia arises because of local bone erosion and because tumors can produce a PTH analogue, PTH-related peptide (PTHrP), and osteoclast-activating cytokines.

Excess vitamin D and other causes

In lymphomas and granulomatous diseases such as sarcoidosis, tuberculosis, and leprosy, macrophages can synthesize vitamin D, which can lead to hypercalcemia. Excess thyroid hormones can increase osteoclast bone resorption, causing hypercalcemia. Adrenocortical insufficiency can cause hypercalcemia. Immobilization causes bone resorption. Rapid bone turnover in Paget's disease can cause hypercalcemia. Excess calcium ingestion as milk and alkali, to relieve peptic ulcer symptoms, causes milk–alkali syndrome with deposition of calcium phosphate. Thiazide diuretics reduce urinary calcium excretion. Mutations in the calcium sensing receptor (CaR) on parathyroid cells cause familial hypocalciuric hypercalcemia.

Clinical features

Mild hypercalcemia is usually asymptomatic. Higher levels cause neurological, gastrointestinal, and renal symptoms ("depressive moans, abdominal groans, renal stones"). There may be drowsiness, lethargy, weakness, depression, and coma. There is often constipation, nausea, vomiting, anorexia, and peptic ulceration. Calcium causes nephrogenic diabetes insipidus, producing dehydration. Sustained hypercalcemia can cause renal stone formation and nephrocalcinosis. Severe chronic hypercalcemia can cause tissue calcification, which may be detectable radiographically or as visible corneal calcification.

ECG changes include *shortening of the Q–T interval*, sometimes with broad T waves and atrioventricular block. Hypercalcemia can potentiate digitalis toxicity.

Treatment

Sodium and water losses should be replaced with intravenous saline to restore body volume and to encourage renal calcium excretion. Loop diuretics can be used to increase the urinary excretion of calcium. Thiazide diuretics should be stopped. Bisphosphonates stabilize bone and inhibit osteoclast action, thus preventing bone resorption. They are useful in malignancy-associated hypercalcemia. Steroids block osteoclast-activating cytokines and are helpful in malignancy and sarcoidosis. If there is excess PTH, surgery to remove parathyroid tissue is often appropriate. In patients with tertiary hyperparathyroidism, calcimimetic drugs can be useful to reduce PTH levels. Calcimimetics, such as cinacalcet, bind the CaR calcium sensor and so inhibit PTH secretion. They also increase the number of vitamin D receptors on the parathyroid cells; vitamin D can act through these receptors to inhibit PTH secretion.

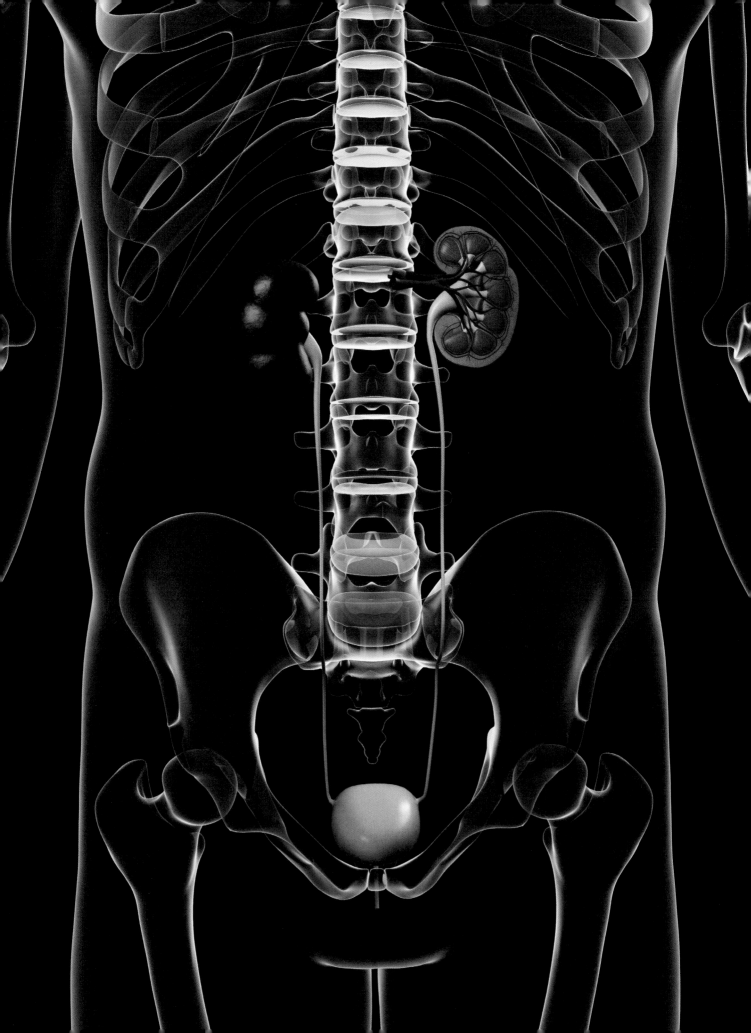

Drugs and genetic disorders

Part 7

Chapters

28 **Drug and organic molecule handling by the kidney** 68
29 **Renal pharmacology: diuretics** 70
30 **Hereditary disorders of tubular transport** 72
31 **Polycystic kidney disease** 74

Don't forget to visit the companion website for this book
www.ataglanceseries.com/renalsystem

28 Drug and organic molecule handling by the kidney

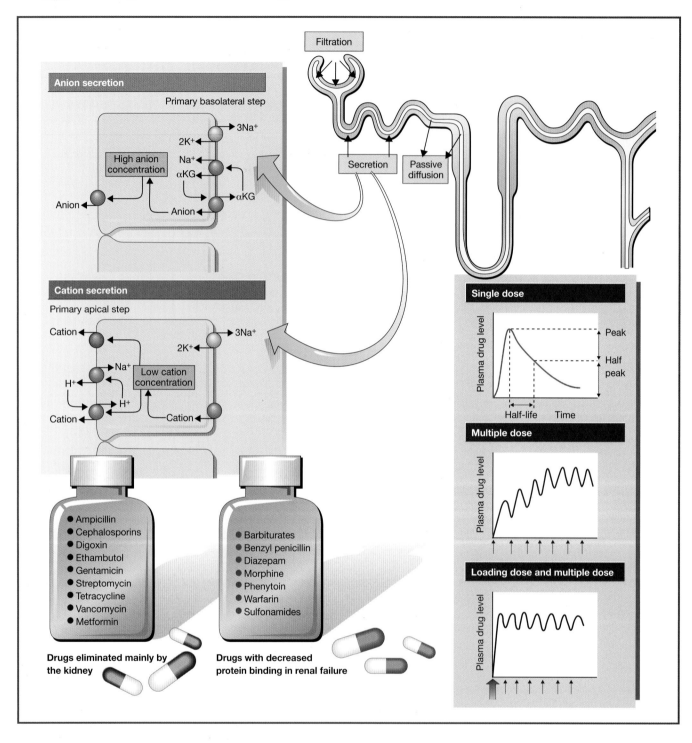

Filtration

Anion secretion

Primary basolateral step

3Na⁺
2K⁺
Na⁺
αKG
αKG
Anion

High anion concentration

Anion

Secretion

Passive diffusion

Cation secretion

Primary apical step

Cation
3Na⁺
2K⁺
Na⁺
H⁺
Low cation concentration
H⁺
Cation
Cation

- Ampicillin
- Cephalosporins
- Digoxin
- Ethambutol
- Gentamicin
- Streptomycin
- Tetracycline
- Vancomycin
- Metformin

Drugs eliminated mainly by the kidney

- Barbiturates
- Benzyl penicillin
- Diazepam
- Morphine
- Phenytoin
- Warfarin
- Sulfonamides

Drugs with decreased protein binding in renal failure

Single dose

Plasma drug level

Peak

Half peak

Half-life   Time

Multiple dose

Plasma drug level

Loading dose and multiple dose

Plasma drug level

Overview of drug kinetics

Unless a drug is injected intravenously, it must be absorbed from its site of administration (usually the gut, skin, or muscle) into the blood and travel to its site of action. Most oral drugs are absorbed in the small bowel. Some drugs undergo "first-pass metabolism" in which they are metabolized or inactivated in the liver, or less commonly in the gut or lung, before they reach the systemic circulation. Once absorbed, a drug equilibrates throughout its volume of distribution, which may include only specific tissues.

The Renal System at a Glance, Fourth Edition. Chris O'Callaghan. © 2017 John Wiley & Sons, Ltd. Published 2017 by John Wiley & Sons, Ltd.
Companion website: www.ataglanceseries.com/renalsystem

Plasma proteins bind many drugs; albumin binds acidic drugs, whereas α_1-acid glycoprotein binds basic drugs. Drugs bound strongly to plasma proteins tend to stay in the circulation. If protein binding is low, the distribution depends on lipid solubility. Water-soluble drugs stay in the extracellular fluid, but lipid-soluble drugs can enter cells and can even be concentrated in adipose tissue.

Drugs can be metabolized, especially in the liver, and the activity of the metabolites may differ from that of the original drug. Phase I reactions cause oxidation, reduction, or hydrolysis of the drug and involve cytochrome P450 mixed function oxidases. Phase II interactions add groups such as glucuronides or sulfates onto phase I products to increase their water solubility. These metabolites may be excreted from the liver in bile or from the kidney in urine. Many drugs are excreted by the kidney, and can accumulate to toxic levels if there is renal impairment.

Renal drug handling

Drugs bound to plasma proteins are not filtered because the proteins are not filtered. Filtration of drugs that are not protein bound depends on their size and charge. Organic anion and cation transporters in the proximal tubule can secrete drugs and are saturable. Tubular reabsorption of drugs is of little importance.

Anions

Basolateral anion transport is fueled by the Na^+/K^+ ATPase. This generates a sodium gradient that drives transport of α-ketoglutarate^{2-} (αKG) into the cell by the sodium dicarboxylate co-transporter (**NaDC3**). Basolateral **OAT** (organic anion transporter) proteins then move anions into the cell in exchange for α-ketoglutarate^{2-}. Anions are transported across the apical membrane by different OAT proteins along concentration gradients.

Cationic drugs do not accumulate in tubular cells because their apical transport out of the cell is actively driven. However, anionic drugs can accumulate to toxic levels because their basolateral transport into the cell is actively driven. Probenecid inhibits the excretion of penicillins by the OAT proteins and has been used to increase plasma penicillin levels.

Cations

Apical cation transport is also fueled by Na^+/K^+ ATPase. This generates a sodium gradient that drives transport of hydrogen out of the cell by the sodium hydrogen exchanger (NHE3). Apical **OCT** (organic cation transporter) proteins then move small cations out of the cell in exchange for hydrogen. There is also active transport of larger cations across by apical membrane by the **MDR1** ATPase transporter. Cations are transported across the basolateral membrane by different OCT proteins along concentration gradients.

Cationic drugs do not accumulate in tubular cells because their apical transport out of the cell is actively driven. However, anionic drugs can accumulate to toxic levels because their basolateral transport into the cell is actively driven. Probenecid inhibits the excretion of penicillins by the OAT proteins and has been used to increase plasma penicillin levels.

Passive diffusion

Lipid-soluble drugs diffuse through cell membranes and across tubular cells. As the urine is concentrated along the nephron, urine drug concentrations increase and lipid-soluble drugs diffuse back into the blood. Water-soluble drugs cannot cross cell membranes and so stay in the urine and are more efficiently excreted by the kidney.

Effect of urine pH

The pH of urine affects whether or not an organic acid or base is protonated and therefore charged. A charge favors water solubility and therefore renal excretion.

Prescribing renally excreted drugs

Renal drug excretion displays first-order kinetics. This means that the rate of drug removal is proportional to the plasma drug concentration. After a single dose, the plasma level rises, peaks, and falls. The half-life is the time taken for the peak level to halve. During steady dosing, it takes around four half-lives to reach a steady state. Administration of a dose equal to the amount of drug in the body at steady state bypasses this delay. A maintenance dose is then half the loading dose given once every half-life. The volume of distribution is calculated by dividing the amount of a drug administered by its plasma concentration. It is the hypothetical volume of plasma that the drug would have to equilibrate into to produce the measured plasma level. Steady-state levels rise with an increase in dose, dose frequency, half-life or drug absorption, and with a fall in the volume of distribution.

Prescribing in renal impairment

Renal impairment reduces glomerular filtration and the tubular secretion of drugs. Drug dosing is usually affected if more than 50% of the normal drug elimination is renal. To avoid toxicity, the dose is reduced or the dosing interval is increased. If necessary, drug levels are monitored. Most polypeptide hormones, including insulin and parathyroid hormone, are metabolized by the kidney and their clearance is reduced in renal impairment. In chronic renal disease, protein binding of acidic drugs (such as phenytoin and theophylline) is reduced because uremic toxins compete for drug-binding sites on albumin. In contrast, protein binding of basic drugs is increased in uremic patients because levels of α_1-acid glycoprotein are elevated.

Dialysis

Water-soluble drugs are better removed by dialysis than lipid-soluble drugs. Heavily protein-bound drugs are poorly removed. A drug such as digoxin, with a very large volume of distribution, has a low plasma concentration and is, therefore, poorly removed. If a drug is mainly eliminated by dialysis, it is usual just to give a dose after each dialysis. Hemofiltration can remove larger molecules than hemodialysis because the membrane pore size is larger in hemofiltration than in hemodialysis. Peritoneal dialysis is relatively inefficient at clearing drugs.

29 Renal pharmacology: diuretics

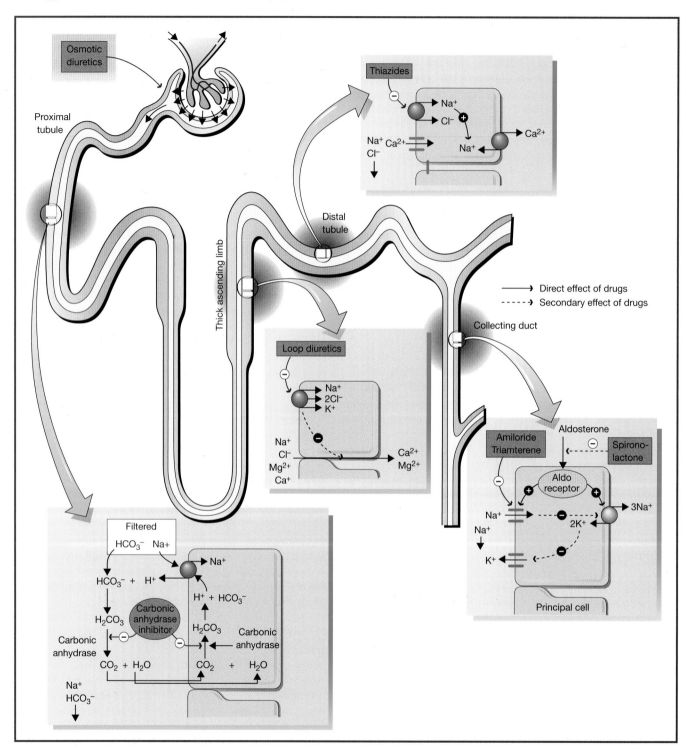

Diuretics increase urine volume. Their action increases the amount of osmotically active substances (usually sodium and chloride ions) in the tubules. This opposes water reabsorption and increases urine volume. Loop diuretics are actively secreted into the tubules by the organic anion transporter (OAT) system (see Chapter 28).

Loop diuretics

Loop diuretics are strong diuretics and include furosemide, bumetanide, and ethacrynic acid. They are highly plasma bound, but are secreted into the tubule by the OAT. They bind the **NKCC2** co-transporter in the thick ascending limb of the loop of Henle. This binding inhibits sodium, potassium, and chloride reabsorption, causing diuresis with loss of these electrolytes. The transcellular voltage difference falls, and paracellular calcium and magnesium reabsorption are also reduced.

Salt reabsorption in the ascending limb normally concentrates the medullary interstitium. By blocking this process, loop diuretics can reduce the ability of the kidney to concentrate urine (see Chapter 11). Increased sodium delivery to the principal cells in the collecting duct increases potassium secretion in return for sodium reabsorption.

Clinical aspects

The relationship between furosemide dose and effect is approximately logarithmic and a small increase in effect requires a large increase in dose. Usually a doubling is required. During long-term use, distal tubule hypertrophy can reduce the efficacy of loop diuretics, and additional inhibition of distal tubule sodium reabsorption by thiazides (especially metolazone) can be useful. This has been termed "serial nephron blockade." In edema states, gut edema impairs absorption of oral furosemide, so intravenous administration can be more effective. Acute intravenous infusion also promotes venodilation, possibly by triggering renal prostaglandin production. Experimentally, loop diuretics reduce energy consumption, helping tubular cells to survive ischemia. However, they do not improve the outcome from renal ischemia in humans.

Adverse effects include sodium, potassium, magnesium, and water depletion. In the long term, plasma and tissue urate levels can rise, triggering gout.

Thiazides: the distal tubular diuretics

Thiazides are generally weak diuretics and are secreted into the proximal tubule. They reversibly inhibit the **NCC** apical NaCl co-transporter in the early distal tubule by binding to the chloride-binding site. More sodium is then delivered to the principal cells of the collecting duct. Some of this excess sodium is exchanged for potassium, causing hypokalemia. Calcium reabsorption is increased and thiazides can be used to treat hypercalciuria. Reduced sodium reabsorption lowers intracellular sodium concentration, promoting basolateral sodium–calcium exchange (via NCX transporters) and therefore calcium reabsorption (see Chapter 25). Thiazides are also used to treat hypertension because they decrease peripheral resistance, but the mechanism of this action is not clear. Secretion of thiazides into the tubules in exchange for urate reabsorption by the OAT system may contribute to raised urate levels.

Adverse effects include sodium, potassium, chloride, and magnesium depletion. Cholesterol and urate levels can rise.

Potassium-sparing collecting duct diuretics

Amiloride and *triamterene* are mainly used to reduce potassium loss caused by loop diuretics. In the principal cells of the cortical collecting duct, sodium entry from the lumen via the ENaC (epithelial sodium channel) is associated with apical potassium exit (see Chapter 17). Sodium reabsorption is therefore linked to potassium secretion and both depend on the activity of the basolateral Na^+/K^+ ATPase. Amiloride competes with sodium for a site in the **ENaC** channel and thus blocks sodium reabsorption and potassium secretion. Triamterene has a similar action.

Aldosterone promotes sodium reabsorption and potassium secretion by increasing transcription of the ENaC channel and the Na^+/K^+ ATPase. *Spironolactone* blocks aldosterone receptors (type 1 mineralocorticoid receptors), so reducing sodium reabsorption and potassium secretion.

Adverse effects of potassium-sparing diuretics include hyperkalemia and, in the case of spironolactone, an antiandrogenic effect that can cause gynecomastia. The antibiotics pentamidine and trimethoprim can cause hyperkalemia by an amiloride-like action.

Carbonic anhydrase inhibitors

Carbonic anhydrase inhibitors block the reaction of carbon dioxide and water and so prevent Na^+/H^+ exchange and bicarbonate reabsorption (see Chapters 19 and 20). The increased bicarbonate levels in the filtrate oppose water reabsorption. Proximal tubule sodium reabsorption is also reduced because it is partly dependent on bicarbonate reabsorption.

Osmotic diuretics

Osmotic diuretics, such as mannitol or glycerol, are filtered in the glomerulus and then not reabsorbed. As the filtrate passes along the nephron, water is reabsorbed, and the concentration of the osmotic diuretic rises until its osmotic effect opposes further reabsorption of water. Sodium is then reabsorbed without water. Eventually, sodium reabsorption is also inhibited because the sodium gradient between filtrate and plasma increases to the point at which sodium leaks back into the lumen.

Mannitol, an osmotic diuretic, draws water from cells osmotically and is used to dehydrate brain cells in cerebral edema. It enhances renal blood flow by increasing extracellular and intravascular volume and reducing red cell volume and blood viscosity. Enhanced blood flow can reduce the medullary interstitial osmolality, reducing the urine-concentrating capacity. Mannitol infusion is sometimes given to prevent acute renal failure in high-risk settings. Its benefit is controversial and excess infusion can cause volume overload if renal function is impaired.

Glucose is filtered in the glomerulus. A high plasma glucose level causes a high filtrate glucose level, which can exceed the tubular capacity for its reabsorption. Glucose then acts as an osmotic diuretic causing volume depletion during diabetic hyperglycemia. High levels of *urea* from protein metabolism can also promote osmotic diuresis in a functioning kidney.

30 Hereditary disorders of tubular transport

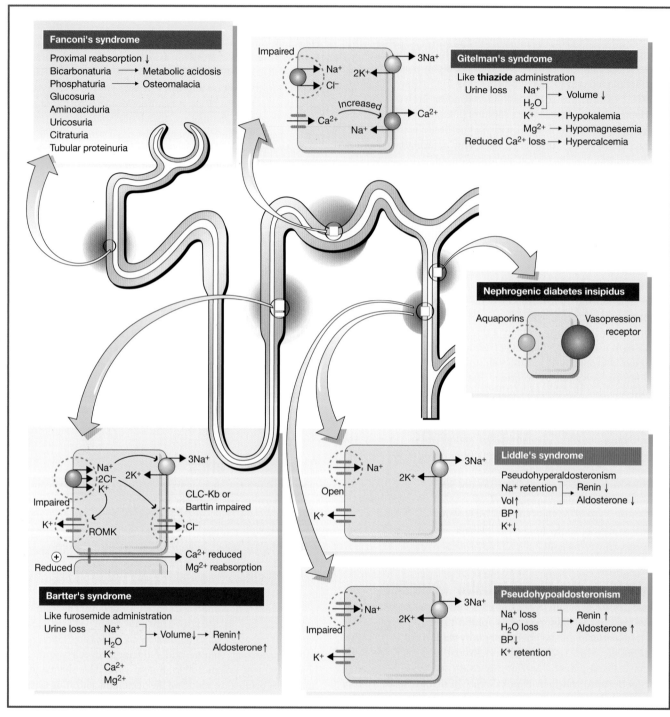

G enetic mutations in the channels involved in sodium, potassium, and chloride handling can produce very similar effects to the diuretic drugs that act on the same channels.

The NKCC2 co-transporter

Mutations that impair the activity of the NKCC2 co-transporter in the thick ascending limb of the loop of Henle cause **Bartter's syndrome**. This condition is characterized by excessive urinary sodium, potassium, and water loss—effects similar to those of furosemide, the diuretic that blocks this channel. The resulting hypokalemia promotes enhanced acid secretion and metabolic alkalosis (see Chapter 21). As the mutant protein cannot transport ions, the transepithelial potential difference falls and the fluid in the tubular lumen loses its positive charge. This reduces calcium reabsorption and causes hypercalciuria, which can predispose to renal stone formation. Renin and aldosterone levels are high to conserve sodium because of volume depletion.

The Renal System at a Glance, Fourth Edition. Chris O'Callaghan. © 2017 John Wiley & Sons, Ltd. Published 2017 by John Wiley & Sons, Ltd.
Companion website: www.ataglanceseries.com/renalsystem

The ROMK and CLC-Kb/barttin channels

Bartter's syndrome can also result from three other mutations affecting ion transport in the thick ascending limb of the loop of Henle—the apical ROMK potassium channel, the basolateral CLC-Kb chloride channel, and barttin, a subunit of mature CLC-Kb chloride channels. Defects in the potassium or chloride channels block the efficient exit of these ions from the cell, and this inhibits the passive entry of sodium, potassium, and chloride into the cell via the NKCC2 transporter. Barttin defects can also cause deafness, as ion transport is important in auditory function.

The NCC sodium/chloride co-transporter

Mutations in the genes encoding the NCC co-transporter in the distal tubule produces **Gitelman's syndrome**. This disorder produces effects similar to those seen with the thiazide diuretics: there is excess loss of sodium, potassium, and magnesium in the urine. The excess urinary potassium loss is the result of enhanced tubular flow, which increases potassium secretion in the cortical collecting duct (see Chapter 16). Hypocalciuria occurs because the inhibition of apical sodium entry into the cell allows intracellular sodium levels to fall, promoting more basolateral sodium/calcium exchange, and therefore more apical calcium entry and greater calcium reabsorption (see Chapters 25 and 29).

The ENaC channels

Different mutations in the ENaC sodium channel in the collecting ducts can switch the channel on or off.

Activating mutations – pseudohyperaldosteronism

These mutations are dominant and leave the ENaC channel open in an unregulated fashion, which causes excess sodium retention, resulting in volume expansion and hypertension and suppressing renin and aldosterone levels. These features constitute **Liddle's syndrome**. Amiloride can be helpful because it blocks the channel. Liddle's syndrome causes pseudohyperaldosteronism by mimicking the effects of aldosterone and causing sodium retention and potassium loss.

Inactivating mutations – pseudohypoaldosteronism

In the ENaC sodium channel, these mutations are recessive and cause excessive sodium loss and potassium retention. These effects promote high renin and high aldosterone levels. The aldosterone cannot exert its effect because of the reduced function of the ENaC channel, with resulting pseudohypoaldosteronism. The condition therefore mimics aldosterone deficiency.

WNK mutations – pseudohypoaldosteronism type 2 (Gordon syndrome)

The WNK1 or WNK4 kinases act on the SPAK and OSR1 kinases to regulate the activity of the NCC co-transporters in the distal tubule. WNK4 causes downregulation of cell surface expression of NCC. Dominant mutations in WNK1 or WNK4 can cause NCC overactivity with excess sodium reabsorption. This reduces the available sodium for sodium/potassium exchange in the distal tubule causing hyperkalemia and metabolic acidosis. The excess sodium reabsorption is associated with hypertension. This condition has the opposite effects to thiazides and so is treated with thiazide diuretics.

Chloride channels and renal stone formation

Mutations in the voltage-gated chloride channels CLC-5 and CLC-Kb cause hypercalciuric nephrolithiasis. CLC-Kb mutations are discussed above. Mutations in CLC-5 Cl^-/H^+ exchanger cause Dent's disease, X-linked recessive hypophosphatemic rickets, and low-molecular-weight proteinuria with hypercalciuria and nephrocalcinosis. These diseases are basically similar and differ mainly in severity. The main features are reduced calcium reabsorption and hypercalciuria, causing renal stone formation, nephrocalcinosis and, in some cases, renal failure. CLC-5 mutations impair the acidification of endosomes involved in proximal tubule endocytic uptake.

Water channels

Nephrogenic diabetes insipidus can result from defects in the aquaporins or the V_2 ADH receptors in the collecting duct (see Chapter 13).

Fanconi's syndrome

There are many inherited and acquired forms of Fanconi's syndrome and only part of the full spectrum of proximal tubular disorders may be present. The major components of Fanconi's syndrome are proximal renal tubular acidosis (caused by reduced bicarbonate reabsorption), glucosuria, aminoaciduria, uricosuria (urinary urate loss) with hypouricemia, citraturia, and phosphate loss with hypophosphatemia and osteomalacia or rickets. There may also be tubular proteinuria as a result of a failure of tubular reabsorption of small proteins and hypokalemia resulting from enhanced distal sodium delivery, which promotes distal potassium secretion. The osmotic load may cause an osmotic diuresis and polyuria.

The syndrome can result from any cause of proximal tubular damage. Causes include vitamin D-dependent rickets caused by defects in the vitamin D_3 receptor or in the renal 1α-hydroxylase enzyme involved in vitamin D synthesis. Metabolic defects in sugar and carbohydrate metabolism, and conditions such as Wilson's disease with abnormal copper deposition, can also cause proximal tubular defects. Cystinosis is a rare condition in which there is excess cystine in the blood; cystine deposition can cause proximal tubular damage. Within the proximal tubule there is active endocytic uptake of proteins including albumin in a process involving the endocytic receptors megalin and cubilin. This process involves acidification of the endosomes by the vacuolar H^+ ATPase. Disruption of these processes can result in proximal tubular dysfunction.

Carbonic anhydrase II deficiency (Guibaud–Vainsel syndrome) impairs bicarbonate reabsorption throughout the nephron, causing both proximal and distal renal tubular acidosis. Defects in the sodium/glucose transporter (SGLT2) in the proximal tubule result in glucosuria. Defects in amino acid reabsorption in the proximal tubule can cause aminoacidurias. The commonest is cystinuria, which results in cystine stone formation (see Chapter 51).

Polycystic kidney disease

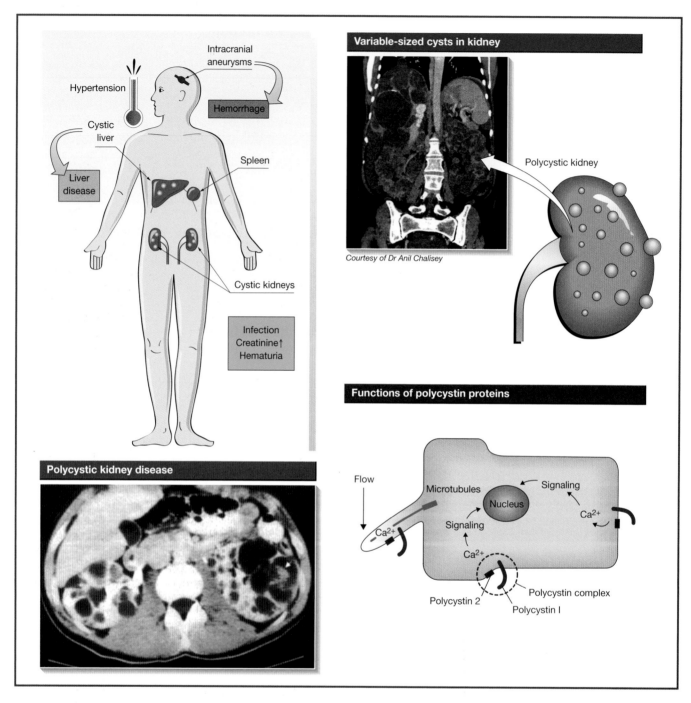

Courtesy of Dr Anil Chalisey

The Renal System at a Glance, Fourth Edition. Chris O'Callaghan. © 2017 John Wiley & Sons, Ltd. Published 2017 by John Wiley & Sons, Ltd.
Companion website: www.ataglanceseries.com/renalsystem

can be asymptomatic, symptoms can result from the presence of the cysts themselves or the effect of the disease on renal function. The cysts can cause pain directly or pain can arise from bleeding into the cysts, infection, or renal stones. High blood pressure is common and may contribute to the reduced life expectancy.

Clinical disease

Renal abnormalities

There are multiple cysts in both kidneys, which can be visualized by ultrasonography, computed tomography (CT), or magnetic resonance imaging (MRI). Cysts vary in size from microscopic to several centimeters in diameter. The cysts are fluid filled and are prone to secondary complications. Distended cysts can cause chronic pain. Bleeding into a cyst can result in acute pain and hematuria. Cysts can become infected and sometimes develop into abscesses.

Renal stone formation is common and may result from urinary stasis, which occurs as a consequence of the cysts. High blood pressure is common and can occur before renal function deteriorates. The reason for this hypertension is not clear. Progressive renal failure is common but does not occur in all patients, and the rate of deterioration varies, even within families. By the age of 50, about 50% of affected individuals have renal failure.

Extrarenal manifestations

Around 50% of patients have cysts in the liver. Although liver function is usually normal, large cysts can cause liver damage and abdominal problems. Cysts in the spleen, pancreas, and other organs are usually asymptomatic. The incidence of intracranial aneurysms is increased over fourfold in ADPKD and these can rupture, resulting in subarachnoid hemorrhage. Noninvasive angiographic screening every 5 years may be of benefit, especially with a family history of aneurysms. A number of patients have cardiac valvular incompetence, especially of the mitral and tricuspid valves. Anemia is less common in patients with renal failure caused by ADPKD than it is in other patients with renal failure because there is sustained erythropoietin production by the kidneys, possibly from the cysts.

Diagnosis

Patients can present with hematuria or pain in the loin or abdomen. More commonly, the diagnosis is made during the investigation of abnormal renal function, hypertension, urinary infection, or stones. There is generally a family history and physical examination may reveal large palpable kidneys (and sometimes liver and spleen) and hypertension. Prenatal diagnosis is now possible for some affected families.

Treatment

There is no specific treatment. High blood pressure and infection should be treated conventionally. If renal failure develops, dialysis or transplantation is required. In animal models, vasopressin antagonists show some benefit. For this reason, it has been suggested that an increased fluid intake of at least 3 L per day may be of benefit as this reduces vasopressin levels. Vasopressin V2 receptor inhibition with tolvaptan has shown some benefit in clinical trials.

Juvenile disease

Although classic ADPKD can manifest itself in children, children can also present with the much more rare autosomal recessive polycystic kidney disease (ARPKD). This is caused by a mutation in the *PKHD1* gene which encodes **fibrocystin**, a membrane protein. This is localized to primary cilia in renal epithelial cells in the collecting duct and in the developing ureteric bud (see Chapter 3).

Molecular pathology

PKD1 and *PKD2*

The *PKD1* gene on chromosome 16 encodes the polycystin-1 protein and the *PKD2* gene on chromosome 4 encodes the polycystin-2 protein. **Polycystin-1** appears to be a membrane receptor capable of interacting with many different molecules and activating a G-protein signaling pathway. **Polycystin-2** is a calcium channel. The two proteins form the **polycystin complex** with other molecules. In renal tubular cells, the complex is found in primary cilia, at cell–cell junctions, and at the points where the cell contacts the extracellular matrix. The complex probably acts as a mechanosensor detecting changes in tubular fluid flow affecting ciliary bending and influencing cellular function accordingly. Bending of the apical primary cilia by fluid flow in the tubule causes entry of calcium into the cell. The extracellular portion of polycystin has many domains that are likely to interact with other molecules and could allow it to detect signals from adjacent cells and from the extracellular matrix. In the adult kidney, polycystin-1 is mainly expressed in the lateral tight junctions in the medullary collecting tubules. However, in the developing kidney, it is also present in the ureteric buds.

Cysts

Cysts arise from any segment of the nephron or collecting duct. They may arise because tubular epithelial cells lose their normal polarization. Certainly, the Na^+/K^+ ATPase that is normally restricted to the basolateral surface of tubular epithelial cells is present on the apical surface of abnormal cystic epithelia. Normal renal tubular cells stop proliferating before birth, but in patients with ADPKD, epithelial cells in cysts continue to proliferate. High levels of epidermal growth factor (EGF) are present in cysts and this promotes proliferation of epithelial cells in the cysts. Analysis of cells isolated from individual cysts has suggested that most cysts are clonally derived, implying derivation from a single cell. As the disease is dominant, affected individuals are heterozygotes, but many cysts are no longer heterozygous, and have lost their normal allele. This suggests that cyst development may require "two hits" from both germline and somatic mutations.

Other cystic diseases

A number of other cystic diseases are caused by mutations in proteins involved in ciliary function. Nephronophthisis is a recessive disease caused by mutations in the nephrocystin gene and results in salt wasting with severe hyponatremia and juvenile kidney failure. Dominant medullary cystic kidney disease, a related disease, is caused by a defect in the *UMOD* gene that encodes uromodulin (Tamm–Horsfall protein) and results in severe salt wasting and adult-onset kidney failure. Different dominant uromodulin mutations cause high urate levels and renal impairment (familial juvenile hyperuricemic nephropathy).

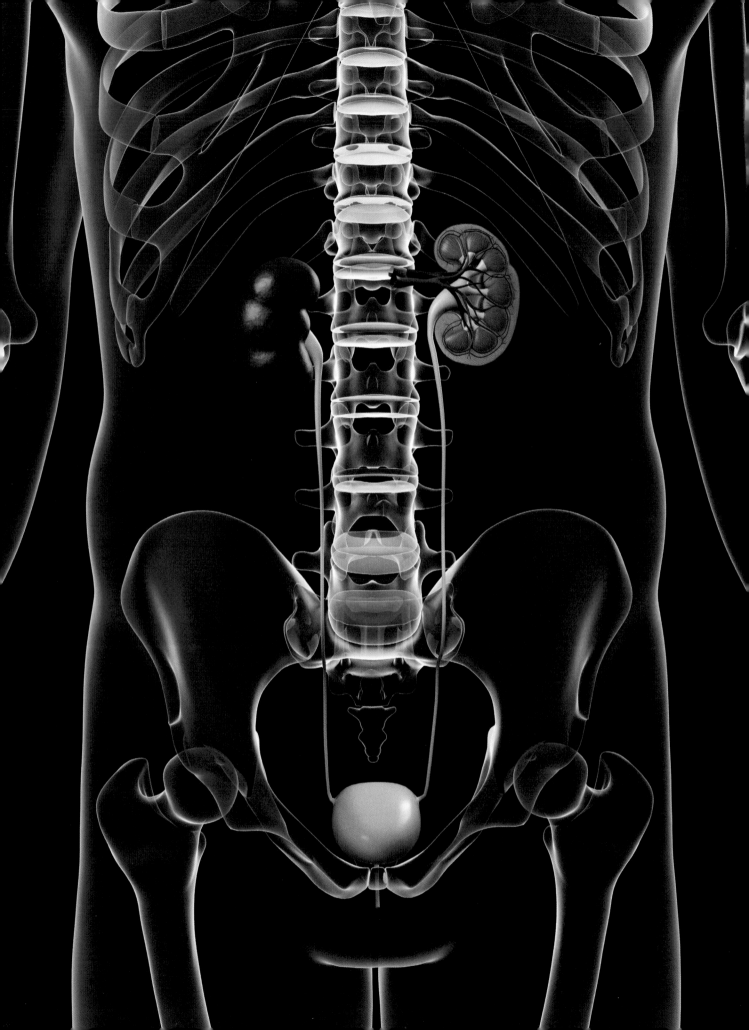

Glomerular and tubulointerstitial disease

Part 8

Chapters

32 Glomerular disease: an overview 78
33 Glomerular pathologies and their associated diseases 80
34 Specific diseases affecting the glomeruli 82
35 Proteinuria and the nephrotic syndrome 84
36 Tubulointerstitial disease 86

Don't forget to visit the companion website for this book
www.ataglanceseries.com/renalsystem

32 Glomerular disease: an overview

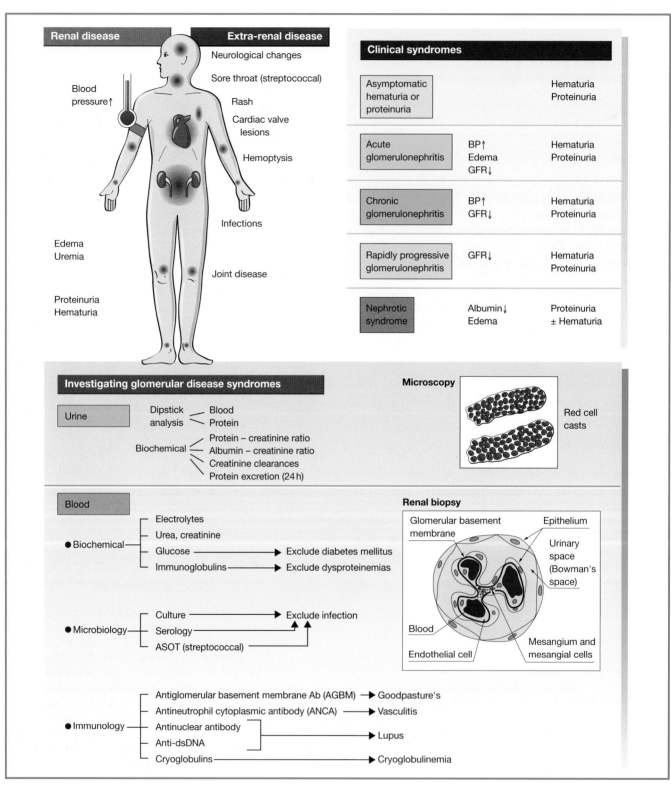

Renal disease

Blood pressure↑

Edema
Uremia

Proteinuria
Hematuria

Extra-renal disease

Neurological changes

Sore throat (streptococcal)

Rash

Cardiac valve lesions

Hemoptysis

Infections

Joint disease

Clinical syndromes

Asymptomatic hematuria or proteinuria		Hematuria Proteinuria
Acute glomerulonephritis	BP↑ Edema GFR↓	Hematuria Proteinuria
Chronic glomerulonephritis	BP↑ GFR↓	Hematuria Proteinuria
Rapidly progressive glomerulonephritis	GFR↓	Hematuria Proteinuria
Nephrotic syndrome	Albumin↓ Edema	Proteinuria ± Hematuria

Investigating glomerular disease syndromes

Urine

Dipstick analysis — Blood
— Protein

Biochemical — Protein – creatinine ratio
Albumin – creatinine ratio
Creatinine clearances
Protein excretion (24 h)

Microscopy

Red cell casts

Blood

● Biochemical — Electrolytes
Urea, creatinine
Glucose → Exclude diabetes mellitus
Immunoglobulins → Exclude dysproteinemias

● Microbiology — Culture → Exclude infection
Serology
ASOT (streptococcal)

● Immunology — Antiglomerular basement membrane Ab (AGBM) → Goodpasture's
Antineutrophil cytoplasmic antibody (ANCA) → Vasculitis
Antinuclear antibody
Anti-dsDNA
Cryoglobulins → Cryoglobulinemia

Lupus

Renal biopsy

Glomerular basement membrane

Epithelium

Urinary space (Bowman's space)

Blood

Endothelial cell

Mesangium and mesangial cells

The Renal System at a Glance, Fourth Edition. Chris O'Callaghan. © 2017 John Wiley & Sons, Ltd. Published 2017 by John Wiley & Sons, Ltd.
Companion website: www.ataglanceseries.com/renalsystem

Although many different diseases act on the glomeruli, the effects of glomerular damage are relatively similar whatever the cause.

- **Reduced glomerular filtration** rate resulting from damage to glomerular components.
- **Proteinuria** caused by protein leakage through the glomerular basement membrane.
- **Hematuria** resulting from active glomerular injury, causing glomerular bleeding.
- **Hypertension** caused by sodium and water retention, often with excess renin secretion.
- **Edema** also resulting from sodium and water retention, often with excess renin secretion.

Classification of glomerular disease

Glomerular disease is primary if only the kidney is affected and secondary if the disease process also affects other tissues. Glomerular disease produces the different clinical syndromes discussed below, such as asymptomatic hematuria or the nephrotic syndrome. Glomerular disease can be classified according to the clinical syndrome produced, the histopathological appearance, or the underlying disease. Only the last is a diagnosis, but the clinical syndrome and histopathological appearances guide the diagnosis. If the etiology is unknown, the histopathological description, such as minimal change disease, also serves as the diagnosis, which is really idiopathic minimal change disease.

Pathological classification

In **proliferative** disease, there is abnormal proliferation of cells within the glomerulus. In severe cases, proliferation of cells, especially macrophages within Bowman's capsule, causes an appearance known as a crescent. In **mesangial** disease, there is excess production of mesangial matrix. In **membranous** disease, the glomerular basement membrane is damaged and thickened. **Membranoproliferative** disease causes both thickening of the glomerular basement membrane and cellular proliferation, usually of mesangial cells. **Vasculitis** is inflammation of the blood vessels. Usually, renal biopsies are interpreted with light microscopy, immunostaining studies and, if necessary, electron microscopy.

- **Focal** disease affects only some glomeruli.
- **Diffuse** disease affects all the glomeruli.
- **Segmental** disease affects only part of the glomerulus.
- **Global** disease affects the whole glomerulus.

Clinical syndromes

Glomerular disease produces five major clinical syndromes. These result from different combinations of the possible effects of glomerular injury. **Asymptomatic proteinuria or hematuria** can result from mild glomerular damage. **Acute glomerulonephritis** is the same as **acute nephritic syndrome** and consists of hematuria, an acute fall in glomerular filtration rate (GFR), sodium and water retention, and hypertension. **Chronic glomerulonephritis** consists of slow progressive glomerular damage, often with proteinuria, hematuria, and hypertension. **Rapidly progressive glomerulonephritis** is a syndrome of very rapid renal failure. There is oliguria and often hematuria and proteinuria, usually without the other features of the nephritic syndrome. **Nephrotic syndrome** consists of heavy proteinuria, leading to hypoalbuminemia and edema (see Chapter 35).

Diagnosing glomerular disease
Clinical assessment

A history of recurrent frank hematuria 1–2 days after an upper respiratory infection suggests IgA nephropathy. Nephritic syndrome occurring 1–3 weeks after an infection suggests postinfective glomerulonephritis, typically poststreptococcal. Hemoptysis with rapidly progressive glomerulonephritis suggests Goodpasture's syndrome. Other features such as skin or joint involvement suggest an underlying condition such as systemic lupus erythematosus or vasculitis. Examination may reveal hypertension, edema, or signs of uremia. It is important to examine for skin, joint, lung, and heart lesions, as well as for neurological disturbances which can indicate systemic lupus erythematosus, vasculitis, or even infection. Both systemic lupus erythematosus and infective endocarditis can cause cardiac valve lesions and glomerular disease. Obesity is associated with focal segmental glomerulosclerosis.

Investigations

Analyze urine for blood and protein, and examine it with a microscope. Red cell casts indicate active glomerular injury causing glomerular bleeding. Measure serum albumin and quantify any proteinuria with a 24-h urine collection or spot urine protein/creatinine ratio or spot albumin/creatinine ratio. Assess GFR from serum urea and creatinine and, if necessary, creatinine clearance. Selected blood tests may indicate a specific diagnosis.

- Blood glucose, immunoglobulins, and blood cultures may indicate diabetes mellitus, myeloma, or other tumors and infection.
- Significant plasma levels of antiglomerular basement membrane (AGBM) antibody indicate antiglomerular basement membrane (Goodpasture's) disease.
- Significant levels of antineutrophil cytoplasmic antibodies (ANCA) suggest systemic vasculitis. If ANCA antibodies are present, these can be checked for specificity against myeloperoxidase (MPO) or protease 3 (PR3).
- Antinuclear antibodies with specificity for double-stranded DNA and low complement levels indicate systemic lupus erythematosus.
- Antibodies against the PLA2R (phospholipase A2 receptor) protein are associated with idiopathic membranous nephropathy.
- Cryoglobulins are present in cryoglobulinemia.
- Lung function tests may be abnormal if there is pulmonary hemorrhage (Goodpasture's syndrome) because blood in the alveoli absorbs the carbon monoxide used to measure gas transfer, which spuriously raises the gas transfer coefficient.

Unless the diagnosis is clinically obvious, a renal biopsy is usually performed.

33 Glomerular pathologies and their associated diseases

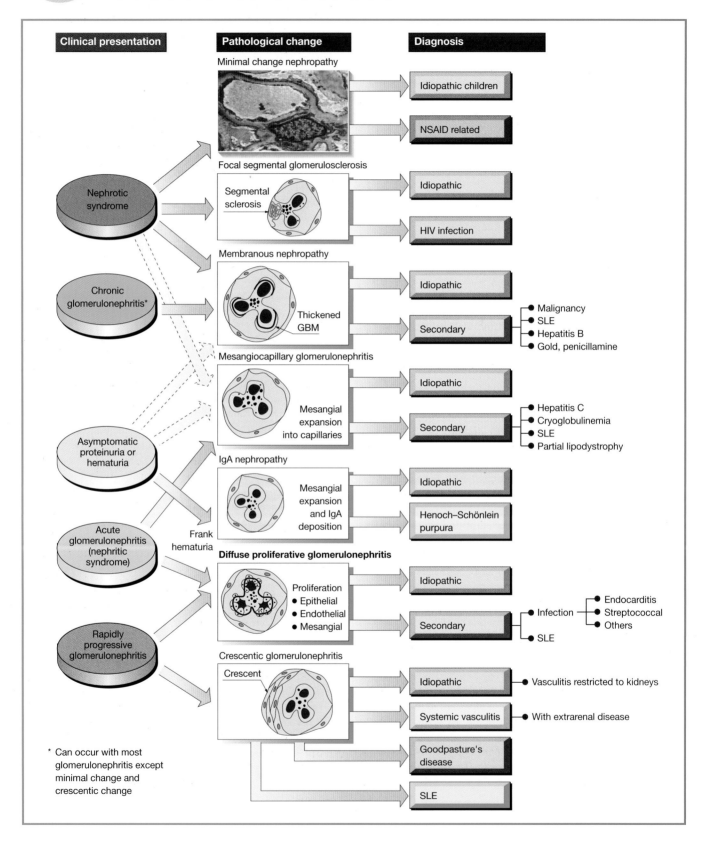

Clinical presentation

- Nephrotic syndrome
- Chronic glomerulonephritis*
- Asymptomatic proteinuria or hematuria
- Acute glomerulonephritis (nephritic syndrome)
- Rapidly progressive glomerulonephritis

Frank hematuria

Pathological change

Minimal change nephropathy

Focal segmental glomerulosclerosis
- Segmental sclerosis

Membranous nephropathy
- Thickened GBM

Mesangiocapillary glomerulonephritis
- Mesangial expansion into capillaries

IgA nephropathy
- Mesangial expansion and IgA deposition

Diffuse proliferative glomerulonephritis
- Proliferation
  - Epithelial
  - Endothelial
  - Mesangial

Crescentic glomerulonephritis
- Crescent

Diagnosis

- Idiopathic children
- NSAID related

- Idiopathic
- HIV infection

- Idiopathic
- Secondary
  - Malignancy
  - SLE
  - Hepatitis B
  - Gold, penicillamine

- Idiopathic
- Secondary
  - Hepatitis C
  - Cryoglobulinemia
  - SLE
  - Partial lipodystrophy

- Idiopathic
- Henoch–Schönlein purpura

- Idiopathic
- Secondary
  - Infection
    - Endocarditis
    - Streptococcal
    - Others
  - SLE

- Idiopathic — Vasculitis restricted to kidneys
- Systemic vasculitis — With extrarenal disease
- Goodpasture's disease
- SLE

* Can occur with most glomerulonephritis except minimal change and crescentic change

The Renal System at a Glance, Fourth Edition. Chris O'Callaghan. © 2017 John Wiley & Sons, Ltd. Published 2017 by John Wiley & Sons, Ltd.
Companion website: www.ataglanceseries.com/renalsystem

Diseases of the glomerular basement membrane

Minimal change nephropathy

Minimal change nephropathy accounts for 90% of the nephrotic syndrome in children and 20% in adults. In children, it is associated with atopy (asthma, eczema, and hay fever), and it often follows an upper respiratory tract infection. The disease is termed "minimal change nephropathy," because light microscopy and immunostaining are normal. However, electron microscopy shows fusion of the podocyte foot processes. The condition responds to steroids and, if it relapses, ciclosporin is useful. Renal impairment does not occur. Nonsteroidal anti-inflammatory drugs can cause minimal change disease.

Focal segmental glomerulosclerosis

This accounts for 15% of the adult nephrotic syndrome and can also cause hematuria and hypertension. Focal and segmental scarring is seen, and the scars contain immunoglobulins and complement. Electron microscopy shows podocyte foot process fusion as in minimal change nephropathy. The two conditions may be different results of an essentially similar disease process. Some patients respond to steroids, which are often given for 4–6 months and relapse may be reduced by ciclosporin or cyclophosphamide. Many patients eventually develop end-stage renal failure and the disease can recur after renal transplantation. A variant is associated with HIV infection and termed HIV-associated neprhopathy (HIVAN). Obesity is now a recognized cause of focal segmental glomerulosclerosis. Defects in the CD2AP slit pore protein have been associated with focal segmental sclerosis in some black patients.

Membranous nephropathy

Membranous nephropathy is the most common cause of the nephrotic syndrome in older patients. There is proteinuria and often renal impairment. Histologically, there is thickening of the glomerular basement membrane and **subepithelial deposits**. It is usually idiopathic, but can be secondary to malignancy, hepatitis B, systemic lupus erythematosus, or use of gold or penicillamine drugs. Idiopathic membranous nephropathy is associated with the presence of autoantibodies against the PLA2R phospholipase A2 receptor in blood and in deposits in the glomeruli. Some patients respond to steroids and chlorambucil or cyclophosphamide, but a minority develop end-stage renal disease.

Proliferative glomerulopathy

Mesangiocapillary glomerulonephritis

This is also known as membranoproliferative glomerulonephritis. It is uncommon and occurs mainly in young adults and children. The presentation varies from asymptomatic hematuria or proteinuria to the usual presentation with combined nephrotic and nephritic syndromes. Most patients develop end-stage renal failure and there is no useful treatment. There is mesangial cell proliferation, excess mesangial matrix, and thickening of the glomerular basement membrane. Most cases are of type 1 with **subendothelial and mesangial immune deposits**. In the more rare type 2 disease, there are immune deposits in the membrane. Type 1 disease is usually associated with systemic lupus erythematosus, infection, or cryoglobulinemia. Patients have low levels of C3 and C4 as a result of complement depletion. Type 2 disease is associated with antibodies that activate and deplete complement, and some patients have the rare disorder partial lipodystrophy.

Immunoglobulin A (IgA) nephropathy (Berger's disease)

Worldwide, this is the most common primary glomerular disease. The typical presentation is in a young man who develops macroscopic hematuria 1–2 days after an upper respiratory tract infection. It can also present with asymptomatic microscopic hematuria, proteinuria, and renal impairment. There is mesangial cell proliferation, increased mesangial matrix, and IgA deposition in the mesangium. Patients often have raised serum IgA levels. Treatment is usually unsuccessful. Nearly a third of patients eventually develop end-stage renal disease and recurrence can occur after renal transplantation.

Henoch–Schönlein purpura

This disease mainly affects children aged under 10. Typically, there is a purpuric rash on the ankles, buttocks, and elbows, abdominal pain, and renal disease. There is usually hematuria, proteinuria, hypertension, fluid retention, and renal impairment, sometimes with the nephrotic syndrome. The histology looks the same as IgA nephropathy. Most children recover fully without treatment.

Diffuse proliferative glomerulonephritis (diffuse endocapillary proliferative glomerulonephritis)

This pathological appearance is typical of **postinfective glomerulonephritis**, which often follows streptococcal infection but can follow other infections, especially infective endocarditis. The classic presentation is nephritic syndrome occurring several weeks after infection. Most patients have low complement levels. There is endothelial and mesangial cell proliferation and glomerular infiltration by neutrophils and monocytes. There is deposition of complement, IgM and IgG on the basement membrane and in the mesangium. Electron microscopy shows **subepithelial deposits**. Antibiotics are given to eradicate any lingering infection and only a few percent of patients develop end-stage renal disease.

Crescentic glomerulonephritis

Crescents are accumulations of macrophages within Bowman's capsule and indicate severe glomerular injury. There are many causes, especially antiglomerular basement membrane disease (Goodpasture's syndrome), systemic vasculitis, and systemic lupus erythematosus, IgA nephropathy, Henoch–Schönlein disease, vasculitis, and cryoglobulinemia. "Idiopathic rapidly progressive glomerulonephritis" may be a form of limited vasculitis.

34 Specific diseases affecting the glomeruli

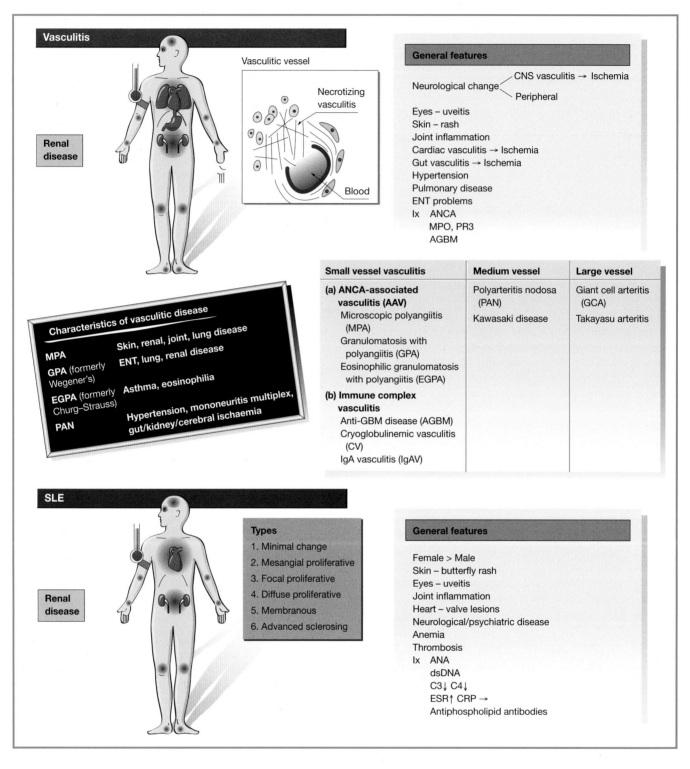

Vasculitis

Vasculitic vessel

Necrotizing vasculitis

Renal disease

Blood

General features

Neurological change — CNS vasculitis → Ischemia
— Peripheral

Eyes – uveitis
Skin – rash
Joint inflammation
Cardiac vasculitis → Ischemia
Gut vasculitis → Ischemia
Hypertension
Pulmonary disease
ENT problems
Ix   ANCA
      MPO, PR3
      AGBM

Characteristics of vasculitic disease

MPA	Skin, renal, joint, lung disease
GPA (formerly Wegener's)	ENT, lung, renal disease
EGPA (formerly Churg–Strauss)	Asthma, eosinophilia
PAN	Hypertension, mononeuritis multiplex, gut/kidney/cerebral ischaemia

Small vessel vasculitis	Medium vessel	Large vessel

(a) ANCA-associated vasculitis (AAV)
  Microscopic polyangiitis (MPA)
  Granulomatosis with polyangiitis (GPA)
  Eosinophilic granulomatosis with polyangiitis (EGPA)
(b) Immune complex vasculitis
  Anti-GBM disease (AGBM)
  Cryoglobulinemic vasculitis (CV)
  IgA vasculitis (IgAV)
	Polyarteritis nodosa (PAN)
	
	Kawasaki disease
		Giant cell arteritis (GCA)
		
		Takayasu arteritis

SLE

Renal disease

Types
1. Minimal change
2. Mesangial proliferative
3. Focal proliferative
4. Diffuse proliferative
5. Membranous
6. Advanced sclerosing

General features

Female > Male
Skin – butterfly rash
Eyes – uveitis
Joint inflammation
Heart – valve lesions
Neurological/psychiatric disease
Anemia
Thrombosis
Ix   ANA
      dsDNA
      C3↓ C4↓
      ESR↑ CRP →
      Antiphospholipid antibodies

Antiglomerular basement membrane disease (Goodpasture's syndrome)

This disease is caused by antibodies against the C-terminal end of the α_3 chain of type 4 collagen in the glomerular basement membrane and the alveolar basement membrane in the lung. The antibody binds to these membranes, triggering inflammation. This causes a vasculitis with rapidly progressive crescentic glomerulonephritis which can lead to acute renal failure and lung hemorrhage. Patients are usually male with the tissue type HLA-DRB1*1501 (usually abbreviated to HLA-DR15). If untreated,

The Renal System at a Glance, Fourth Edition. Chris O'Callaghan. © 2017 John Wiley & Sons, Ltd. Published 2017 by John Wiley & Sons, Ltd.
Companion website: www.ataglanceseries.com/renalsystem

patients die from pulmonary hemorrhage or renal failure. Treatment involves plasma exchange to remove the antibodies and immunosuppression with steroids and cyclophosphamide to inhibit glomerular inflammation and reduce antibody production. If treated early, most patients recover and relapse is uncommon.

Primary systemic vasculitis

The primary vasculitic diseases produce necrotizing inflammation of vessels and often affect the kidneys, respiratory tract, joints, skin, and nervous system. They are classified according to the size of the predominant vessels affected and the presence or absence of granulomata (see figure). Small vessel ANCA-associated vasculitis (AAV) includes microscopic polyangiitis (MPA), granulomatosis with polyangiitis (GPA, formerly Wegener's granulomatosis), and eosinophilic granulomatosis with polyangiitis (EGPA, formerly Churg–Strauss syndrome). ANCA-associated vasculitis can cause a focal segmental proliferative glomerulonephritis with necrosis and crescent formation. Clinically, this often presents as rapidly progressive glomerulonephritis. Histologically, there is infiltration of the glomeruli by neutrophils, but no complement or immunoglobulin deposition. Antineutrophil cytoplasmic antibodies (ANCA) against neutrophil granule contents are usually, but not always, present. Patients with GPA have a cytoplasmic or **c-ANCA** reactivity against proteinase 3. Patients with MPA have a perinuclear or **p-ANCA** reactivity against myeloperoxidase. Renal disease is more common with MPA and GPA then with EGPA. Therapy is initially with steroids and cyclophosphamide. After several months, azathioprine may be substituted for the cyclophosphamide. Plasma exchange is sometimes used in the acute phase. **Idiopathic rapidly progressive glomerulonephritis** is a small vessel single organ vasculitis (SOV) affecting only the kidneys. There is no ANCA, but it is treated like the other small vessel disorders.

Systemic lupus erythematosus

This is a multisystem disease which can affect the nervous system, joints, skin, kidneys, and heart. The renal effects vary and have been classified by the World Health Organization and modified by the International Society of Nephrology as: type 1 – minimal change on light microscopy; type 2 – mesangial proliferative; type 3 – focal proliferative; type 4 – diffuse proliferative; type 5 – membranous; and type 6 – advanced sclerosing. The renal presentation depends on the histological lesion. It is typically nephrotic syndrome or renal impairment and can be acute. There are usually antinuclear antibodies to double-stranded DNA and low complement levels. Typically, the ESR (erythrocyte sedimentation rate) is raised. A raised CRP (C-reactive protein) indicates infection. Treatment for renal disease with steroids and cyclophosphamide or azathioprine is usually helpful. Plasma exchange is sometimes used.

Cryoglobulinemia

Cryoglobulins are immunoglobulins that precipitate in the cold and may cause a small vessel cryoglobulinemic vasculitis (CV). They occur in inflammatory or neoplastic diseases, including myeloma, lymphoma, multisystem autoimmune diseases, and chronic infection. Plasma complement levels are usually low. Typically, cryoglobulins cause a type 1 mesangiocapillary glomerulonephritis. Mixed essential cryoglobulinemia is usually caused by hepatitis C infection. The clinical presentation is usually of a purpuric vasculitic rash, arthralgia, peripheral neuropathy, and glomerulonephritis. Cryoglobulins are removed by plasma exchange in severe disease.

Dysproteinemias

These disorders are characterized by excess antibody production by benign or malignant plasma cell activity. Malignant disease or myeloma can cause various renal problems, including glomerular deposition of amyloid fibrils, tubular toxicity from filtered light chains, which may form casts in the tubules (myeloma cast nephropathy), and mesangiocapillary glomerulonephritis resulting from glomerular deposition of light chains (light chain deposition disease). The presence of free immunoglobulin light chain (Bence Jones protein) in the urine or a monoclonal band in plasma raises the possibility of myeloma.

Rheumatoid arthritis and connective tissue diseases

Rheumatoid arthritis can cause renal amyloid deposition, mesangial proliferative glomerulonephritis, membranous nephropathy, or a focal segmental glomerulonephritis with vasculitis and necrosis. Systemic sclerosis or scleroderma is rarely associated with a crescentic glomerulonephritis. More commonly, there is hyperplasia of small renal arteries. Any additional vasospasm causes acute renal ischemia. This "renal crisis" triggers renin release, which worsens the vasospasm and promotes severe hypertension.

Amyloidosis

Amyloid protein is usually a combination of amyloid P protein with either antibody light chains (AL amyloid) or the inflammatory amyloid A protein (AA amyloid). AL amyloid is typical of dysproteinemias, whereas AA amyloid is typical of chronic inflammatory diseases. Amyloid deposition can damage the kidney, liver, spleen, heart, tongue, and nervous system. Amyloidosis can cause proteinuria and nephrotic syndrome. Histologically, amyloid proteins can be visualized by Congo red or immunostaining in the glomeruli, the tubules, and the blood vessels. Treatment aims to reduce production of the amyloid proteins by treating any underlying dysproteinemia or inflammatory disease.

Drug causes of glomerular disease

Gold and penicillamine can both cause membranous nephropathy. Hydralazine causes a lupus-like disease. Nonsteroidal anti-inflammatory drugs can cause minimal change glomerular disease, with nephrotic syndrome and sometimes with an interstitial nephritis.

Hereditary and other causes of glomerular disease

Thin basement membrane disease causes asymptomatic microscopic hematuria. The condition is inherited and does not normally cause renal deterioration. Alport's disease is usually an X-linked mutation in the α_5 chain of type 4 collagen, a component of the glomerular basement membrane. It causes proteinuria, hematuria, renal failure, and sensorineural deafness.

35 Proteinuria and the nephrotic syndrome

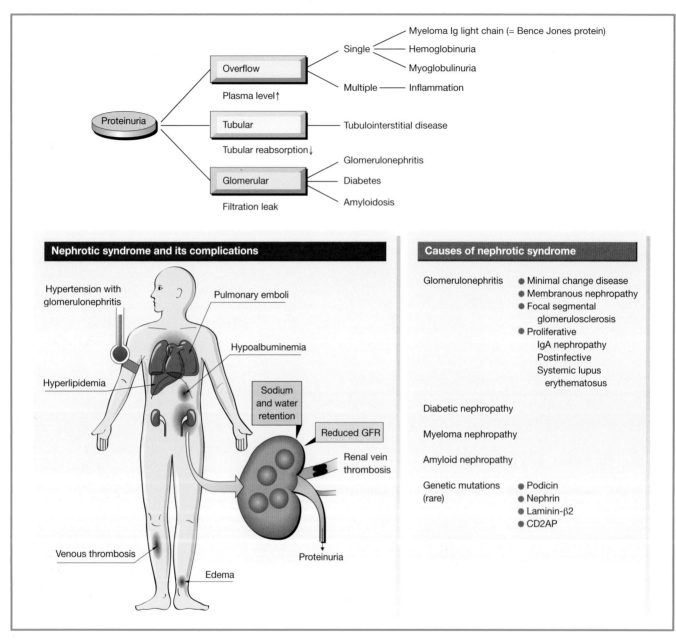

Clinically detectable proteinuria is abnormal and is usually an early marker of renal disease. The nephrotic syndrome occurs when proteinuria is severe enough to cause hypoalbuminemia and there is associated sodium and water retention, causing edema. All causes of nephrotic proteinuria result in abnormal foot processes consistent with defects in the slit diaphragm and the size selectivity of filtration. Congenital nephrotic syndrome in children can result from defects in the slit membrane proteins nephrin and podocin, the glomerular basement membrane protein laminin-β_2 and the CD2AP protein. In many renal diseases there are high levels of angiotensin II, which can downregulate nephrin, causing disruption of slit membrane structure and proteinuria. Mutations in the actin-binding proteins α-actinin-4 or INF2 can cause congenital focal segmental glomerulosclerosis as can mutations in WT1 and phospholipase C-epsilon-1. Mutations in the TRPC6 calcium channel gene can cause focal segmental glomerulosclerosis. APOL1 gene variants contribute to a high rate of focal segmental glomerulosclerosis in African-Americans.

Types of proteinuria

Plasma proteins are filtered at the glomerulus according to their size and charge. Small proteins of less than 20 kDa are freely

The Renal System at a Glance, Fourth Edition. Chris O'Callaghan. © 2017 John Wiley & Sons, Ltd. Published 2017 by John Wiley & Sons, Ltd.

Companion website: www.ataglanceseries.com/renalsystem

filtered, then reabsorbed, and degraded in the proximal tubule. Reabsorption involves uptake by the endocytic receptors megalin and cubilin. This process catabolizes hormones, such as insulin, and small immunological molecules, such as immunoglobulin light chains. Therefore, isolated loss of small proteins in the urine (**selective proteinuria**) indicates either *overflow proteinuria* (caused by excess serum and filtered protein levels overwhelming normal tubular reabsorption), or *tubular proteinuria* (resulting from impaired tubular reabsorption). The filtration barrier is normal. Large proteins such as albumin, transferrin, and IgG are not normally filtered and are lost in urine only if the glomerular filtration barrier is damaged. This relatively **nonselective proteinuria** is termed *glomerular proteinuria*.

Proteinuria is detected with urine dipsticks and can be quantified with a 24-h urine collection or spot urine. Proteinuria in the nephrotic range is >3.5 g/24 h or on a spot urine the protein: creatinine ratio is above 350 mg/mmol or 40 mg/mg or g/g. Assessment of albumin in urine is more reliable than measurement of total urine protein content, particularly at lower levels of proteinuria. A urine albumin:creatinine ratio (ACR) of >3 mg/mmol (>30 mg/g) indicates abnormal protein loss consistent with early chronic kidney disease. An ACR of >30 mg/mmol (>300 mg/g) represents a substantial protein leak and this may reach >220 mg/mmol in nephrotic syndrome. The ACR is used to detect very low levels of albuminuria in early diabetic nephropathy. **Urinary protein electrophoresis** can distinguish different types of proteinuria. With tubular and overflow proteinuria, only low-molecular-weight proteins are present. With overflow proteinuria, there is generally one abundant protein in the urine, typically an immunoglobulin light chain resulting from a B-cell disorder such as myeloma. Rarely, inflammation can cause overflow of many small acute-phase proteins. Glomerular proteinuria is dominated by albumin because of its high plasma concentration and there are lesser amounts of transferrin and IgG.

Clinical features of the nephrotic syndrome

Nephrotic patients usually present with edema. Their urine may be frothy because of its high protein content. The most common causes are minimal change glomerulonephritis in children and membranous nephropathy or focal segmental glomerulosclerosis in adults (see Chapter 33). A prothrombotic state, hypertension, and hyperlipidemia all contribute to a higher incidence of ischemic heart disease in nephrotic patients. Unless there is obvious diabetic nephropathy or clinically typical childhood minimal change glomerulonephritis, a histological diagnosis is made by renal biopsy.

Renal sodium retention and edema

Hypoalbuminemia may reduce intravascular volume leading to renal hypoperfusion and renin-mediated hyperaldosteronism (see Chapter 15).

Protein loss, malnutrition, and infection

Urinary protein loss can cause negative protein balance and protein malnutrition. Patients have a tendency to infection, possibly because IgG and other immune proteins are lost in urine. Pneumococcal infection was a particular problem, but the use of pneumococcal vaccine and prophylactic antibiotics have reduced this.

Thrombosis

Thromboregulatory proteins, such as antithrombin III, protein S, and protein C, are lost in urine, and hypoproteinemia increases liver synthesis of fibrinogen, raising fibrinogen levels. These changes promote venous thrombosis, especially in the renal and deep leg veins. Pulmonary emboli can then occur. Renal vein thrombosis can cause a sudden deterioration in renal function with flank pain and hematuria.

Hyperlipidemia

There is increased hepatic lipid and apolipoprotein synthesis and reduced chylomicron and very-low-density lipoprotein (VLDL) catabolism. These changes may result in urinary loss of liporegulatory substances and cause a rise in plasma LDL cholesterol and VLDL. Hyperlipidemia requires diet and drug therapy, usually with a statin.

Renal impairment

Glomerular filtration is often reduced and nephrotic kidneys are vulnerable to prerenal acute renal failure. Disruption of the normal arrangement of epithelial foot processes probably reduces the number of functional interpodocyte filtration slits. Although each slit is highly permeable, there may be a reduction in the total surface area for filtration and so a fall in glomerular filtration rate (GFR).

Treatment

Any underlying renal disease process, such as a glomerulonephritis, should be treated if appropriate. Both minimal change disease and focal segmental glomerulosclerosis may respond to a course of steroids. A renal biopsy is usually performed in adults, but children are often given a course of steroids without a biopsy as the most likely cause is minimal change nephropathy (see Chapter 33). Some general measures may also be useful. Angiotensin-converting enzyme (ACE) inhibitors or angiotensin receptor blockers (ARBs) often reduce proteinuria, possibly by blocking a direct effect of angiotensin II on the filtration barrier. Nonsteroidal anti-inflammatory drugs such as indomethacin reduce the GFR, filtration fraction, and proteinuria, but can worsen sodium retention and trigger acute renal failure. Both ACE inhibitors and nonsteroidal anti-inflammatory drugs can cause hyperkalemia. In extreme cases, renal embolization or nephrectomy has been performed to prevent severe proteinuria. Edema can be treated with sodium restriction and diuretics (see Chapter 15). Prophylactic support stockings and heparin or warfarin can help to prevent thrombosis with severe proteinuria or hypoalbuminemia.

Pregnancy and proteinuria

Proteinuria can also occur during pregnancy, especially from systemic lupus erythematosus. However, in the last trimester of pregnancy, pre-eclampsia can cause hypertension, edema, and proteinuria. If protein loss is high, nephrotic syndrome can result (see Chapter 39).

36 Tubulointerstitial disease

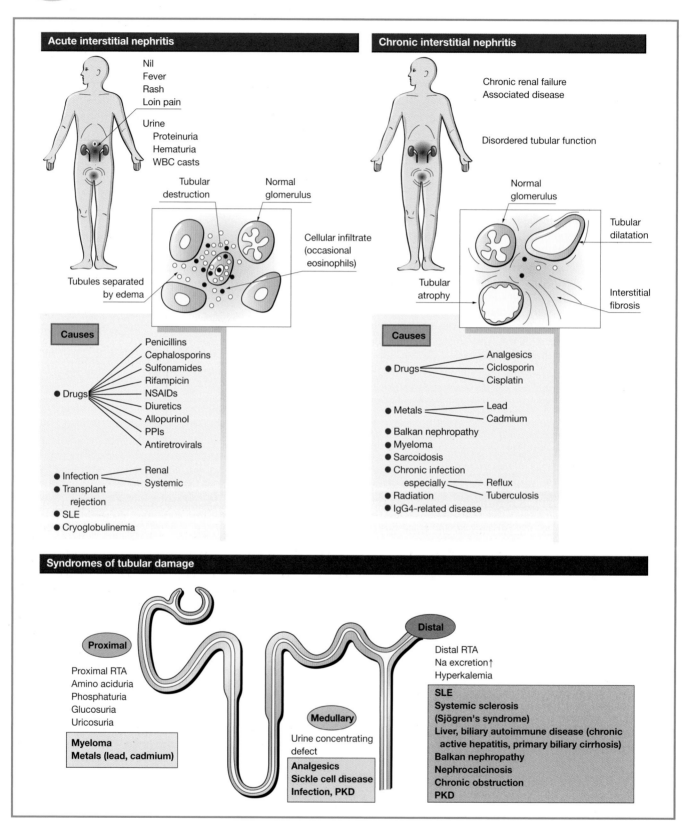

Acute interstitial nephritis

Nil
Fever
Rash
Loin pain

Urine
Proteinuria
Hematuria
WBC casts

Tubular destruction
Normal glomerulus
Cellular infiltrate (occasional eosinophils)
Tubules separated by edema

Causes

- Drugs
  - Penicillins
  - Cephalosporins
  - Sulfonamides
  - Rifampicin
  - NSAIDs
  - Diuretics
  - Allopurinol
  - PPIs
  - Antiretrovirals
- Infection
  - Renal
  - Systemic
- Transplant rejection
- SLE
- Cryoglobulinemia

Chronic interstitial nephritis

Chronic renal failure
Associated disease

Disordered tubular function

Normal glomerulus
Tubular dilatation
Tubular atrophy
Interstitial fibrosis

Causes

- Drugs
  - Analgesics
  - Ciclosporin
  - Cisplatin
- Metals
  - Lead
  - Cadmium
- Balkan nephropathy
- Myeloma
- Sarcoidosis
- Chronic infection especially
  - Reflux
  - Tuberculosis
- Radiation
- IgG4-related disease

Syndromes of tubular damage

Proximal

Proximal RTA
Amino aciduria
Phosphaturia
Glucosuria
Uricosuria

**Myeloma
Metals (lead, cadmium)**

Medullary

Urine concentrating defect

**Analgesics
Sickle cell disease
Infection, PKD**

Distal

Distal RTA
Na excretion↑
Hyperkalemia

**SLE
Systemic sclerosis
(Sjögren's syndrome)
Liver, biliary autoimmune disease (chronic active hepatitis, primary biliary cirrhosis)
Balkan nephropathy
Nephrocalcinosis
Chronic obstruction
PKD**

The Renal System at a Glance, Fourth Edition. Chris O'Callaghan. © 2017 John Wiley & Sons, Ltd. Published 2017 by John Wiley & Sons, Ltd.
Companion website: www.ataglanceseries.com/renalsystem

The tubules and the renal interstitium are in intimate contact and are both affected by a range of disease processes. The clinical presentation is determined by the effect on tubular function. Typically, the tubules either become blocked, which reduces glomerular filtration, or their transport functions become impaired, which reduces water and solute reabsorption. Important presentations of tubulointerstitial damage are acute and chronic interstitial nephritis. Interstitial changes also occur in acute tubular necrosis, acute renal transplant rejection, and urinary tract obstruction. Certain diseases, mainly hereditary, impair tubular function without causing interstitial changes.

Acute interstitial nephritis

This causes acute diffuse renal inflammation and there can be a rapid deterioration in renal function. Acute interstitial nephritis is usually asymptomatic but, if it is drug induced, there may be a maculopapular rash, fever, or eosinophilia. Lumbar pain can occur, probably as a result of stretching of the renal capsule. There may be mild proteinuria, microscopic hematuria, white blood cell casts, and eosinophils in the urine. Ultrasonography usually shows slightly enlarged kidneys. Formal diagnosis requires a renal biopsy. There is infiltration of the interstitium with inflammatory cells, particularly monocytes and T cells. The tubular basement membrane may be disrupted and tubules may be compressed by the infiltrating cells. Treatment involves discontinuation of any drug that could be the cause, treatment of any infection, and often immunosuppression with steroids. The prognosis is good.

Etiology of acute interstitial nephritis

The main cause is an allergic reaction to a drug, particularly **nonsteroidal anti-inflammatory drugs** (NSAIDs), proton pump inhibitors (PPIs) such as omeprazole, allopurinol, diuretics, antiretroviral drugs (e.g., tenofovir, indinavir), 5-aminosalicylates (e.g., mesalamine/mesalazine), and antibiotics (especially penicillins, cephalosporins, rifampicin [rifampin], and sulfonamides). Systemic or renal infection, typically acute pyelonephritis, can cause an acute interstitial nephritis. Gout causes excess urate excretion and urate crystals can precipitate in the tubules, causing tubular obstruction and triggering inflammation.

Chronic interstitial nephritis

Typically, this presents as either chronic renal failure or with symptoms of an associated primary disease. Hypertension is common, the glomerular filtration rate (GFR) is reduced, and there is mild proteinuria, microscopic hematuria, and inflammatory cells in the urine. Tubular transport and reabsorption can be impaired, resulting in features such as glycosuria. Destruction of interstitial erythropoietin-producing cells can cause anemia. Tubular cells are flat and atrophic, the tubules are dilated, and there is interstitial fibrosis with a mononuclear cell infiltrate.

Etiology of chronic interstitial nephritis

Antibody light chains are filtered in the glomerulus and normally reabsorbed in the proximal tubule by receptor-mediated endocytosis. In **myeloma**, the high level of light chains saturates this reabsorption leading to light chain excretion (Bence Jones proteinuria). Light chains are toxic to tubules and cause tubular inflammation and damage (see Chapter 34). Excess use of **analgesics** such as aspirin, paracetamol (acetaminophen), and **NSAIDs** (and in the past, phenacetin) causes chronic interstitial nephritis and sometimes papillary necrosis. **Other causes** of chronic interstitial nephritis include excess lead or cadmium intake, radiation, sarcoidosis, IgG4-related disease, and Balkan nephropathy (an endemic chronic interstitial disease affecting countries around the Balkan sea and probably caused by exposure to dietary aristolochic acid).

Papillary necrosis

The medulla receives all its blood supply from the vasa recta, which makes the papillae highly vulnerable to ischemic damage and hypoxia. In addition, the counter-current system concentrates some toxins, such as analgesics, in the medulla and papillae. If there is severe medullary ischemia or interstitial damage, the function of the loop of Henle and collecting ducts may be impaired. In the worst cases, damaged papillae can slough off and even obstruct the ureters. Causes include analgesic use, diabetes mellitus, infection, and sickle-cell disease. In sickle-cell disease, medullary ischemia promotes red blood cell sickling in the papillae. In diabetes mellitus, infection and vascular disease promote ischemic papillary damage.

Disorders of tubular function

Disorders of tubular function include aminoacidurias, renal tubular acidoses, Bartter's syndrome, vitamin D-resistant rickets, nephrogenic diabetes insipidus, and Fanconi's syndrome (see Chapters 13, 24, 27, and 30). There are three main patterns of tubular damage which reflect the transport functions of the damaged tubule segment. The abnormalities of tubular function can occur alone in specific diseases or as part of acute or more usually chronic tubulointerstitial nephritis.

Proximal tubule damage impairs proximal tubular reabsorption. Possible consequences include aminoaciduria, glycosuria, phosphaturia, uricosuria, and bicarbonaturia leading to metabolic acidosis (proximal renal tubular acidosis). Low molecular weight proteinuria can also arise due to disruption of the normal endocytic uptake of filtered proteins by the proximal tubules (see Chapter 2).

Distal tubule damage can impair distal bicarbonate reabsorption and aldosterone-regulated sodium reabsorption, and the related potassium secretion. The bicarbonaturia causes metabolic acidosis (distal renal tubular acidosis).

Medullary damage affects the loop of Henle and collecting ducts, reducing the kidneys' ability to concentrate urine. This can occur after infection, analgesic use, and sickle-cell disease, and in the polyuric recovery phase of acute tubular necrosis.

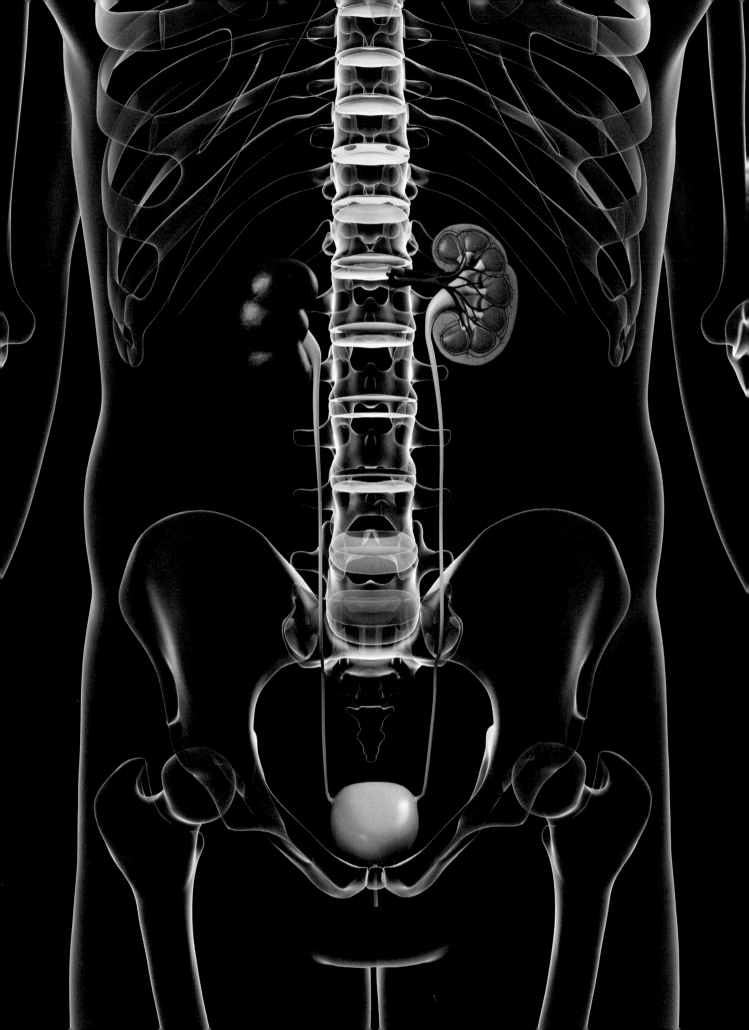

Systemic conditions and the renal system

Part 9

Chapters

37 Hypertension: causes and clinical evaluation   90
38 Hypertension: complications and therapy   92
39 Pregnancy and the renal system   94
40 Diabetes mellitus and the kidney   96

Don't forget to visit the companion website for this book
www.ataglanceseries.com/renalsystem

37 Hypertension: causes and clinical evaluation

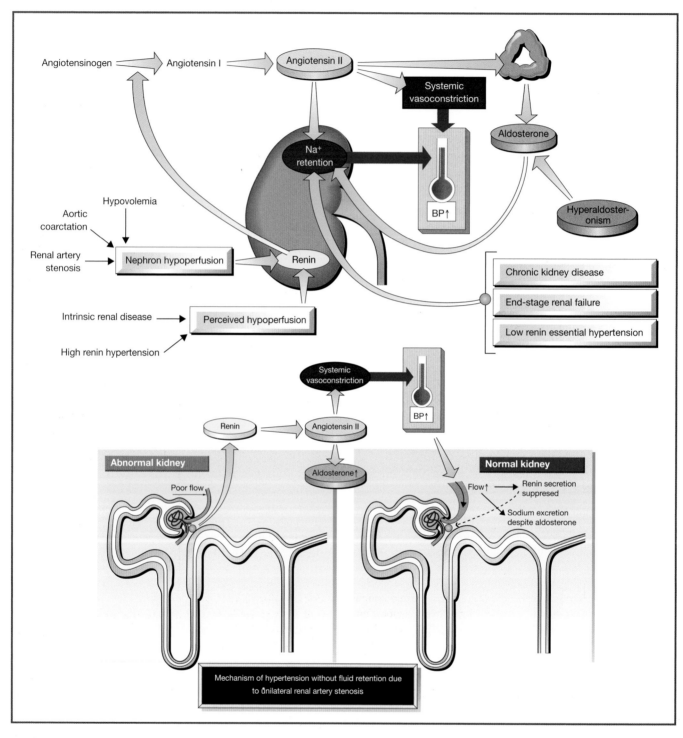

Mechanism of hypertension without fluid retention due to unilateral renal artery stenosis

Hypertension is defined as blood pressure greater than 140/90 mm Hg. It can damage vessels and organs and increases mortality. Treatment improves the prognosis. If a cause is identified, hypertension is said to be secondary; if there is no identifiable cause, it is termed primary or essential hypertension. Blood pressure is determined by cardiac output, systemic vascular resistance, and circulatory volume. The key determinant of systemic vascular resistance is vasoconstriction of arterioles and the key determinant of circulatory volume is renal sodium handling. Genome-wide analyses in essential hypertension implicate multiple genes, including some involved in the kidney (e.g., uromodulin), ion transporters (e.g., the NBC sodium-bicarbonate co-transporter), endothelial function (e.g., nitric oxide synthase), natriuretic peptides, and the renin–angiotensin–aldosterone system.

The Renal System at a Glance, Fourth Edition. Chris O'Callaghan. © 2017 John Wiley & Sons, Ltd. Published 2017 by John Wiley & Sons, Ltd.
Companion website: www.ataglanceseries.com/renalsystem

Causes of secondary hypertension

Renal artery stenosis

Renal artery stenosis (see Chapter 8) reduces renal blood flow and the glomerular filtration rate (GFR), stimulating renin release and angiotensin II production. Angiotensin II causes hypertension by vasoconstriction and stimulation of aldosterone release and sodium retention. If both kidneys are affected, the hypervolemia and hypertension eventually restore renal perfusion and renin levels fall slightly. If only one kidney is normal, the hypertension increases its GFR. This promotes sodium excretion by the healthy kidney, but the stenosed kidney remains underperfused and continues to produce very high renin levels.

Primary hyperaldosteronism

Primary hyperaldosteronism accounts for 1–2% of all hypertension. Excess aldosterone increases renal sodium retention and potassium secretion. The resulting hypervolemia causes hypertension. Renin production is suppressed because renal perfusion pressure and sodium chloride delivery to the macula densa are increased.

Intrinsic renal disease

Any renal disease can cause hypertension. Severe renal impairment reduces sodium excretion and causes hypervolemia and hypertension, which is "salt sensitive" because it is increased by salt intake. With milder renal impairment, perceived renal hypoperfusion promotes renin secretion and angiotensin II-mediated vasoconstriction. This hypertension is not salt sensitive and is termed salt resistant.

Defects in tubular sodium handling

Pseudohypoaldosteronism type 2 due to WNK1 or WNK4 mutations causes distal tubular NCC sodium chloride co-transporter overactivity with excess sodium retention, hyperkalemia, and hypertension (see Chapter 30). Liddle's syndrome of pseudohyperaldosteronism also causes excess sodium retention, hypokalemia, and hypertension.

Other causes of hypertension

Coarctation of the aorta reduces renal perfusion and triggers renin secretion. Characteristically, pulses are weaker in the legs than in the arms. **Steroids** cause sodium retention and hypertension. This is a mineralocorticoid effect of administered and endogenous glucocorticoids. **Catecholamine** release by a pheochromocytoma causes vasoconstrictive hypertension. **Drugs** can cause hypertension, especially steroids, ciclosporin, and estrogens in oral contraceptives. **Obesity** is often associated with hypertension.

Pathogenesis of primary hypertension

Essential or primary hypertension is characterized by an increase in peripheral resistance. This can be caused by two mechanisms which may coexist.

High renin/salt resistant/dry essential hypertension

These patients have raised renin levels for their body sodium content. This causes angiotensin II release with vasoconstriction, aldosterone secretion, and sodium retention. However, the filtration fraction and sodium excretion increase to a greater extent and the patient can become hypovolemic. The hypertension is salt resistant because salt excretion is not impaired. The excess angiotensin II causes vasoconstriction and also promotes vascular smooth muscle hypertrophy and proliferation. High renin and angiotensin II levels in hypertension correlate with vascular and end-organ damage. High angiotensin II levels may downregulate nephrin in the glomerulus, leading to proteinuria. Mild hypovolemia may cause mild tissue ischemia. High renin hypertension responds best to inhibition of the renin–angiotensin II axis with **angiotensin-converting enzyme inhibitors**, **angiotensin receptor blockers**, or **β-blockers** (which inhibit renin secretion).

Low renin/salt sensitive/wet essential hypertension

These patients have renal sodium and water retention, which suppress renin secretion. The hypertension worsens with a high salt intake. Sodium retention may be caused by increased sympathetic adrenergic activity or a defect in sodium-coupled calcium transport. Excess sodium may cause vasoconstriction by altering smooth muscle calcium fluxes. Patients respond to **sodium restriction**, **diuretics**, α_1-**adrenergic blockers**, and **calcium channel antagonists**. People of African ethnicity typically have this pattern of hypertension.

Clinical evaluation of hypertension

Hypertension is diagnosed if blood pressure is consistently raised above 140/90 on at least three separate occasions or is above 135/85 on 24-h ambulatory blood pressure monitoring. A large cuff must be used with a large arm, otherwise a falsely high reading will be obtained. The beginning of the first sound indicates the systolic pressure and the end of the last sound the diastolic pressure. Hypertensive retinopathy confirms the presence of hypertension and may indicate malignant hypertension. Hypertension is often associated with obesity, excess alcohol intake, insulin resistance, and gout. Baseline investigations include urinalysis, a full blood count, serum electrolytes, lipid profile and glucose (preferably fasted), and electrocardiography (ECG), ideally with echocardiography to identify left ventricular hypertrophy. Hypokalemia suggests primary hyperaldosteronism. Further investigations may include uric acid, plasma and urinary catecholamine, or vanillylmandelic acid (VMA) levels to exclude pheochromocytomas, adrenal function tests to check for steroid excess, and renal angiography to exclude renal artery stenosis.

Paired plasma renin and aldosterone levels can be useful in the presence of hypertension and hypokalemia. If both are raised, this suggests secondary hyperaldosteronism, such as that caused by high renin levels in renal artery stenosis (see Chapter 8). If the renin is low and the aldosterone is high, that suggests primary hyperaldosteronism. However, if both are low, then there may be another explanation for the apparent mineralocorticoid activity such as high glucocorticoid levels. Treatment with ACE inhibitors, AngII receptor blockers or diuretics can elevate the ratio of renin to aldosterone, but a very low or undetectable renin level raises the suspicion of primary hyperaldosteronism.

38 Hypertension: complications and therapy

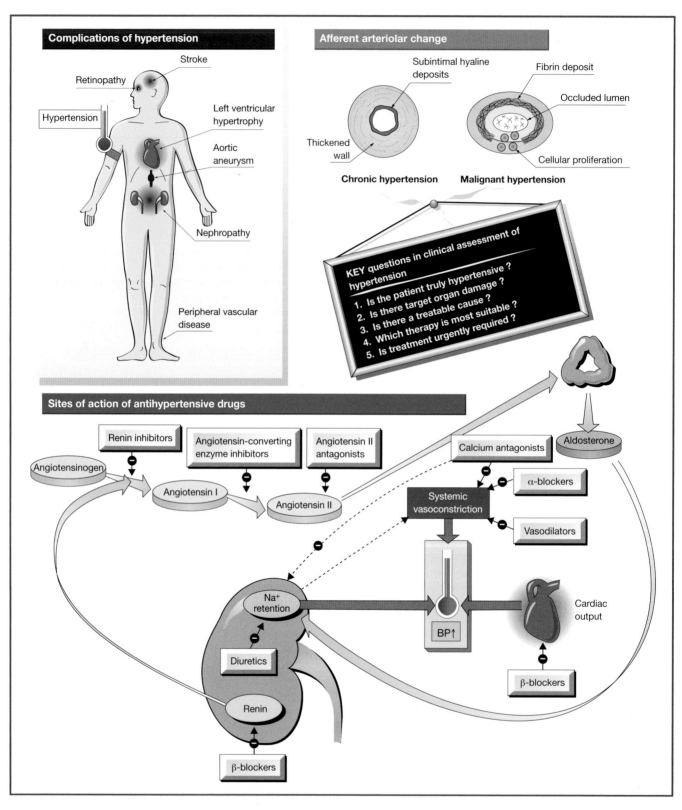

Complications of hypertension

Stroke
Retinopathy
Hypertension
Left ventricular hypertrophy
Aortic aneurysm
Nephropathy
Peripheral vascular disease

Afferent arteriolar change

Subintimal hyaline deposits
Thickened wall
Chronic hypertension

Fibrin deposit
Occluded lumen
Cellular proliferation
Malignant hypertension

KEY questions in clinical assessment of hypertension

1. Is the patient truly hypertensive ?
2. Is there target organ damage ?
3. Is there a treatable cause ?
4. Which therapy is most suitable ?
5. Is treatment urgently required ?

Sites of action of antihypertensive drugs

Renin inhibitors
Angiotensin-converting enzyme inhibitors
Angiotensin II antagonists
Calcium antagonists
Aldosterone
α-blockers
Vasodilators

Angiotensinogen
Angiotensin I
Angiotensin II
Systemic vasoconstriction

Na⁺ retention
Diuretics
Renin
β-blockers

BP↑
Cardiac output
β-blockers

Complications of hypertension

Renal complications

Microalbuminuria and dipstick proteinuria are early signs of hypertensive nephropathy. Blood pressure control slows the rate of renal damage. The groups most likely to develop hypertensive renal damage are elderly people, obese individuals, black patients, and those from the Indian subcontinent, especially those with diabetes. The primary insult is damage to the renal vessels from the raised pressure. In the interlobular artery walls, muscle is replaced by sclerotic tissue. The afferent arteriole walls undergo hyalinization—the subintimal deposition of lipids and glycoproteins exuded from plasma. Damage to these resistance vessels exposes the glomerular capillary endothelium to damaging hypertension. This reduces glomerular blood flow and filtration, and promotes proteinuria. Inflammatory proteins are exuded from the plasma and ultimately there is glomerular sclerosis or ischemic atrophy.

Cardiovascular complications

The high vascular resistance strains the heart, causing left ventricular hypertrophy. Hypertension also increases the atherosclerosis of arteries.

Retinopathy

Retinopathy is common and is graded according to severity. Grade 3 or 4 indicates accelerated or "malignant" hypertension. **Grade 1**—arterial spasm, tortuous arteries, silver-wire appearance. **Grade 2**—arteriovenous nipping. Veins appear narrowed as arteries pass over them. **Grade 3**—hemorrhage, including flame hemorrhage. Lipid extravasation causes exudates; hard exudates are old, but soft exudates or cotton-wool spots indicate acute severe hypertension. **Grade 4**—papilledema. A swollen optic disc.

Malignant or accelerated hypertension

This is severe hypertension with grade 3 or 4 retinal changes and renal damage. It can arise anew or as a complication of essential or secondary hypertension. The central feature is renal vessel damage, usually caused by hypertension. This damage reduces renal blood flow, triggering renin secretion, which promotes further hypertension and sodium retention. Damage to the endothelium can cause fibrinoid necrosis—fibrin enters the vessel wall, triggering cellular proliferation, vessel occlusion, and ischemia.

The clinical presentation can be of headache, visual disturbance, or shortness of breath as a result of cardiac problems. Renal impairment is common, often with hematuria and proteinuria. Damaged vessels can harm red blood cells, causing a microangiopathic hemolytic anemia. **Treatment** is with angiotensin-converting enzyme (ACE) inhibitors, angiotensin receptor blockers, or β-blockers to block the renin cycle. Care is required because patients may have renal artery stenosis (see Chapter 8). Diuretics promote sodium excretion. Hypertensive encephalopathy, pulmonary edema, or severe acute renal disease may require intravenous treatment with sodium nitroprusside, hydralazine, labetalol, or a nitrate preparation.

Treatment of hypertension

Unless there is severe hypertension, end-organ damage, or malignant hypertension, treatment is not urgent. Blood pressure may be improved by exercise, reduced alcohol consumption, and correction of obesity, increased fruit and vegetable intake, and reduced total and saturated fat intake. A reduction in salt intake is recommended, especially if there is renal impairment (see Chapter 37). Other risk factors for vascular disease, such as hyperlipidemia, should be modified when possible. Treatment aims to reduce clinic blood pressure measurements to <140/90 (<150/90 in the elderly) or ambulatory or home monitored blood pressure to <135/80 (<145/85 in the elderly). There are adverse effects of hypertensive therapy and impotence in men can be a reason for poor compliance. If treatment of hypertension is not effective it can be useful to monitor blood pressure for several hours after supervised ingestion of the prescribed medication.

- **ACE inhibitors** inhibit angiotensin II production. They reduce intraglomerular pressure by dilating efferent arterioles more than afferent arterioles. This reduces proteinuria and glomerulosclerosis. Complications include hyperkalemia caused by reduced aldosterone production and renal impairment if renal artery stenosis is present. ACE degrades bradykinin, so ACE inhibitors cause high bradykinin levels that can cause cough.
- **Angiotensin II receptor blockers** (ARBs), such as losartan, are antagonists and have the same effect as ACE inhibitors. Cough is not a problem.
- **β-blockers** suppress renin secretion, reduce cardiac output, and may have a centrally mediated effect. Lowering the cardiac output can worsen the symptoms of peripheral vascular disease. β-blockers blunt the catecholaminergic effects that normally warn people with diabetes of hypoglycemia. $β_1$-selective blockers avoid the bronchospasm of $β_2$ blockade.
- **Calcium channel blockers** cause vasodilation. In salt-sensitive hypertension, they also increase sodium excretion by poorly understood mechanisms. Verapamil and diltiazem reduce atrioventricular nodal conduction and should not be given with β-blockers. Nifedipine dilates only afferent arterioles, allowing systemic hypertension to cause intraglomerular hypertension.
- **Diuretics**, mainly thiazides, are used in hypertension, but these are ineffective if the glomerular filtration rate is low. Furosemide may then be beneficial.
- **$α_1$-antagonists**, such as doxazosin, block catecholaminergic vasoconstriction and can cause postural hypotension. However, they improve insulin sensitivity, lipid profiles, and sometimes, erectile function, and can increase urine flow rates when there is prostatic hypertrophy.
- **Direct vasodilators**, such as sodium nitroprusside, intravenous nitrates, hydralazine, diazoxide, and minoxidil, cause peripheral vasodilation directly. This usually results in reflex tachycardia. Prolonged intravenous sodium nitroprusside administration causes toxic thiocyanate concentrations and, after 48 h, levels should be monitored.
- **Centrally acting drugs**, such as clonidine, methyldopa, and guanethidine, are seldom used as a result of multiple side effects. Clonidine and methyldopa result in central $α_2$-receptor agonism which reduces sympathetic activity and lowers vascular resistance, heart rate, and blood pressure.
- **Direct renin inhibitors**, such as aliskiren, are available as treatments for hypertension, but are not widely used.

39 Pregnancy and the renal system

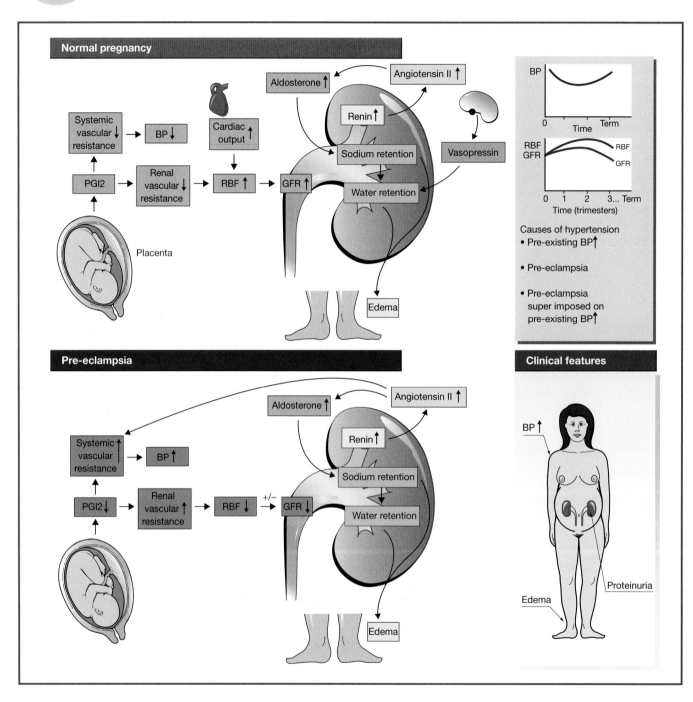

The normal placenta makes prostaglandin **PGI2**, which causes general vasodilation, and **progesterone**, which causes relaxation of connective tissues. In pregnancy, the combination of a rise in cardiac output by up to 40% and renal vasodilation due to PGI2, increases both renal blood flow and glomerular filtration rate. Consequently, creatinine levels are usually low (<80 μmol/L). Renin, angiotensin II, and aldosterone levels all rise, but blood pressure falls because the vasodilating effect of PGI2 overcomes the vasoconstricting influence of angiotensin II. The rise in aldosterone contributes to sodium retention, which promotes retention of around 12–13 kg of water. Thirty to eighty percent of pregnant women have detectable edema. The osmotic thresholds for vasopressin secretion and thirst fall, resulting in a fall of 10 mOsmol/kg H_2O in plasma osmolality and 5 mmol/L in plasma sodium. Plasma volume increases more than total red blood cell volume so hemoglobin levels fall. There is potassium retention, because progesterone overcomes the potassium losing effects of the high aldosterone levels. Pco_2, HCO_3^-, and pH all fall, and a compensated respiratory alkalosis develops (see Chapter 23).

Urinary tract infection (see Chapter 50) in pregnancy is more likely to involve the upper urinary tract, due to reflux up the relaxed ureters. Acute pyelonephritis can result. For this reason pregnant women are screened for asymptomatic bacteriuria, which is treated if identified.

The risk factors for **acute tubular necrosis** are similar to those for nonpregnant women. **Acute cortical necrosis** can occur when sepsis, volume depletion, or other renal insults occur during pregnancy and renal function may not recover. Renal arteriography shows no cortical perfusion. The pathophysiology probably involves intense renal vasoconstriction.

Urate is freely filtered in the glomerulus and then almost completely reabsorbed in the early proximal tubule principally via apical URAT1 transporters and basolateral OAT transporters. Urate secretion in the later proximal tubule determines urate excretion and is proportional to the renal blood flow to the peritubular capillaries. Urate levels are therefore a good index of renal blood flow in pregnancy.

Hypertension

Blood pressure falls during the first trimester, is at its lowest during the second trimester, and then rises toward term. The causes of hypertension in pregnancy are pre-existing chronic hypertension, pre-eclampsia, and pregnancy-induced hypertension. Pre-eclampsia can be superimposed on a background of chronic hypertension. Pregnancy-induced hypertension first occurs during pregnancy, then returns to normal afterward. However, chronic hypertension often develops later and these patients may be early in the pathogenesis of chronic hypertension when hypertension is only manifest under the stress of pregnancy. Blood pressure in pregnancy is generally below 140/90. Raised blood pressure is usually treated as it can reduce placental perfusion and harm the fetus. Drugs that appear safe are methyldopa, labetalol, nifedipine, and alpha blockers such as doxazosin. ACE inhibitors have toxic effects on the fetus, including renal failure.

Pre-eclampsia and eclampsia

Pre-eclampsia typically occurs after 32 weeks, but can occur after 20 weeks or up to 10 days after delivery. Early onset disease is usually most severe. Risk factors include previous pre-eclampsia, a first pregnancy, a multiple pregnancy, obesity, hypertension, diabetes mellitus, renal impairment, and a family history. Pre-eclampsia is characterized by hypertension, proteinuria, and edema. Untreated pre-eclampsia can progress to eclampsia, in which seizures can occur.

In pre-eclampsia, placental dysfunction arises and reduces the production of vasodilating PGI2, allowing unopposed vasoconstrictors, such as angiotensin II, to cause a rise in systemic vascular resistance and hypertension. Renal blood flow falls, further stimulating renin secretion and angiotensin II production. Hypertension is transmitted to the glomerular capillaries causing proteinuria. The effects of angiotensin (and usually norepinephrine or noradrenaline) promote renal sodium retention causing edema. The vasoconstriction reduces renal blood flow, but its effect is greater in the efferent than the afferent arterioles, which helps to maintain the glomerular filtration rate. Therefore, plasma creatinine may not be elevated, but plasma urate rises because its excretion depends on renal blood flow.

The cause of the placental dysfunction is unclear but may involve an immune trigger from the pregnancy that reduces placental perfusion. Pre-eclampsia has been classified into "placental pre-eclampsia" in which the primary defect is placenta development and function and "maternal pre-eclampsia" in which the placenta is initially normal, but primary defects are present in the mother's circulation, such as hypertension, diabetes mellitus, or obesity. The end result in either case is that the maternal–placenta interaction is abnormal and placental function is compromised. The clinical consequence is a systemic illness with dysfunction of the mother's endothelium, which can cause problems in different organs and in the general circulation.

Renal biopsy is not usually performed but may show endothelial cell swelling, mesangial cell proliferation, and fibrin deposition. Variants of eclampsia affecting other systems include the HELLP syndrome (hemolysis, elevated liver enzymes, and low platelets) and acute fatty liver of pregnancy. The treatment of pre-eclampsia involves bed rest in hospital and antihypertensive therapy. Severe pre-eclampsia or eclampsia requires delivery of the baby. Unless there is definite volume depletion, intravenous fluid administration is avoided as it can cause dangerous hypertension and pulmonary edema. In high-risk pregnancies, aspirin is of benefit.

Pre-existing renal disease

Any renal impairment may worsen during pregnancy and the deterioration may not be reversible. Hypertension is common and pre-eclampsia is increased. Both hypertension and renal impairment contribute to miscarriage, intrauterine growth retardation, and superimposed pre-eclampsia. Patients on dialysis have poor fertility and are unlikely to sustain a full pregnancy. Patients with functioning renal transplants often have successful pregnancies, even on immunosuppression.

Systemic lupus erythematosus

In systemic lupus erythematosus (SLE), the pregnancy outcome is better if the disease is in remission and blood pressure and renal function are normal. Puerperal relapse can occur. Anti-phospholipid syndrome can cause abortion, intrauterine growth retardation, thromboembolism, and early onset pre-eclampsia. Anti-Rho antibodies can cause congenital heart block.

40 Diabetes mellitus and the kidney

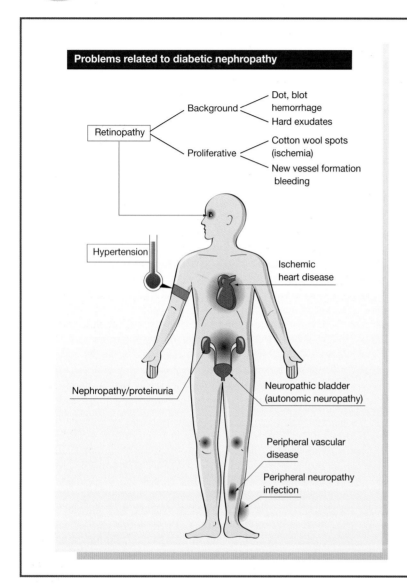

Problems related to diabetic nephropathy

Retinopathy
- Background
  - Dot, blot hemorrhage
  - Hard exudates
- Proliferative
  - Cotton wool spots (ischemia)
  - New vessel formation bleeding

Hypertension

Ischemic heart disease

Nephropathy/proteinuria

Neuropathic bladder (autonomic neuropathy)

Peripheral vascular disease

Peripheral neuropathy infection

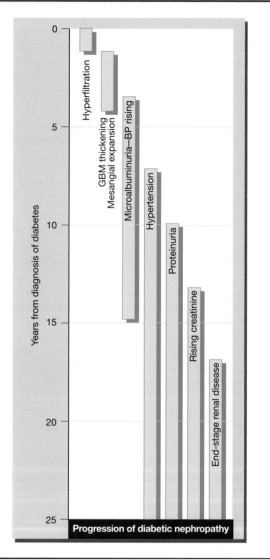

Progression of diabetic nephropathy

Years from diagnosis of diabetes

Hyperfiltration

GBM thickening Mesangial expansion

Microalbuminuria—BP rising

Hypertension

Proteinuria

Rising creatinine

End-stage renal disease

Between 25% and 50% of all patients with diabetes develop nephropathy. Diabetes is the commonest single cause of end-stage renal disease and accounts for 30–40% of all cases.

Clinical progression of diabetic nephropathy

A minority of patients, especially those with poor glycemic control, already have enlarged kidneys with an increased glomerular filtration rate (GFR) at the time that their diabetes is diagnosed. This hyperfiltration may result from intraglomerular hypertension caused by preferential efferent arteriolar constriction. The next renal abnormality to develop is microalbuminuria with an elevated albumin:creatinine ratio (ACR) of >3 mg/mmol (>30 mg/g), which can be below the detection threshold of conventional dipsticks. Microalbuminuria is a strong predictor of subsequent nephropathy and is associated with mild hypertension and mild insulin resistance. After a period of microalbuminuria, patients may progress to overt nephropathy, with hypertension, dipstick proteinuria, ACR >30 mg/mmol (>300 mg/g), and a linear decline in GFR. Severe proteinuria can cause the nephrotic syndrome. Most patients with nephropathy also have retinopathy and hyperlipidemia. If retinopathy is present, a renal biopsy is not usually necessary but, if it is absent, other causes of renal disease, especially renal artery stenosis, should be excluded.

Microvascular changes in diabetic kidneys are typical of diabetic changes occurring elsewhere, such as in the retina. The vessel walls become thickened with glycosylated matrix, and in some cases vessel occlusion develops. These changes impair oxygen diffusion out of the vessel, causing tissue ischemia. In the retina this leads to new vessel formation. In patients with Type 2 diabetes mellitus (noninsulin dependent), nephropathy is less common in those of European descent than in those of

The Renal System at a Glance, Fourth Edition. Chris O'Callaghan. © 2017 John Wiley & Sons, Ltd. Published 2017 by John Wiley & Sons, Ltd.
Companion website: www.ataglanceseries.com/renalsystem

African or Asian descent. It takes about 15–20 years from the onset of proteinuria to develop end-stage renal disease, but many patients with Type 2 diabetes mellitus die before this as a result of cardiovascular disease.

Factors promoting nephropathy in people with diabetes

Good glycemic control has been shown to slow the rate at which proteinuria develops and progresses in Type 1 diabetes mellitus (Diabetes Control and Complications Trial or DCCT) and in Type 2 diabetes mellitus (UK Prospective Diabetes Study or UKPDS). Hyperglycemia causes protein glycosylation, which promotes protein cross-linking. Cross-linking could either interfere with collagen molecules of the glomerular basement membrane or trigger mesangial cells to secrete the excess extracellular matrix that is present. Increased intraglomerular pressure causes early hyperfiltration and may also damage the endothelium and glomerular filtration barrier. Growth-promoting hormones, such as growth hormone, insulin-like growth factor, and platelet-derived growth factors, may promote the early renal hypertrophy and trigger the accompanying renal hemodynamic changes. There is reduced nephrin expression in the slit membrane in patients with Type 1 and Type 2 diabetes mellitus and this could contribute to proteinuria (see Chapters 1 and 35). There is a familial tendency to nephropathy in both Type 1 and 2 diabetes. Candidate genes include the red cell sodium/lithium co-transporter, the red cell sodium/hydrogen counter-transporter, and the angiotensin-converting enzyme (ACE).

Histological changes

The glomerular basement membrane is thickened with deposition of albumin and other plasma proteins within it. There is mesangial expansion causing loss of filtration surface. Afferent and efferent arterioles undergo hyalinosis as a result of the deposition of lipid and glycoprotein material in the arterial wall. Nodular exudative lesions and diffuse glomerulosclerosis represent long-standing nephropathy.

Treatment

Pre-end-stage renal disease

Patients with diabetes should be monitored for microalbuminuria at least once a year. If microalbuminuria is detected, ACE inhibitors have been shown to reduce proteinuria and reduce the probability of progression to end-stage renal disease. Angiotensin receptor blockers are likely to have a similar effect. Angiotensin II can downregulate nephrin protein levels in glomerular filtration slit pores, which may contribute to proteinuria, and ACE inhibitors block this effect. Strict blood pressure control (<130/80 mm Hg)

can also reduce proteinuria and progression to end-stage renal disease. Good glycemic control reduces the probability of microvascular complications such as nephropathy in Type 1 and 2 diabetes. If renal impairment develops in Type 2 diabetes, only short-acting hypoglycemic drugs metabolized by the liver, such as gliclazide and tolbutamide, should be used. Other drugs may accumulate. Metformin, a biguanide, should be stopped with significant renal impairment as it can accumulate and can cause lactic acidosis.

End-stage renal disease

People with diabetes who have end-stage renal disease have a higher mortality than patients who do not have diabetes but have end-stage renal disease, irrespective of the mode of renal replacement therapy. The main causes of death are cardiovascular disease and infection. Renal transplantation offers the best prognosis and quality of life. Some units perform routine coronary angiography and revascularization before renal transplantation because of the high incidence of coronary artery disease. Diabetic foot problems, caused by a combination of peripheral vascular disease, peripheral neuropathy, and infection, are especially common after transplantation and can result in the need to amputate. Combined kidney and pancreas transplantations are increasingly performed in patients who have diabetic nephropathy. Rejection rates are higher than for kidneys alone and more immunosuppression is required, but the quality of life is usually much improved if the transplantation is successful.

The half-life of insulin is increased with severe renal impairment. Insulin requirements fall and there is an increased risk of hypoglycemia. Altered red cell survival on hemodialysis or peritoneal dialysis makes glycated hemoglobin measurements unreliable, and regular home monitoring of glucose is preferable. It is possible to put insulin into peritoneal dialysis bags to provide glycemic control, avoiding subcutaneous injection of insulin. Retinopathy and blindness can affect the patient's ability to perform peritoneal dialysis. Diabetic patients have a high incidence of vascular disease, and the modification of risk factors for vascular disease, such as hyperlipidemia, is important.

Other renal problems related to diabetes

Diabetes can contribute to papillary ischemia, especially if there is also infection or abuse of analgesics. The result is papillary necrosis (see Chapter 36) with sloughing of the papilla and often hematuria and pyuria. Urinary tract infection is more common in people with diabetes and a contributory factor can be incomplete voiding of urine, resulting from autonomic neuropathy. Diabetic renal damage can reduce renin levels, causing hypoaldosteronism with consequent hyperkalemia, sodium loss, and metabolic acidosis (see Chapter 24). This is sometimes termed a type 4 renal tubular acidosis.

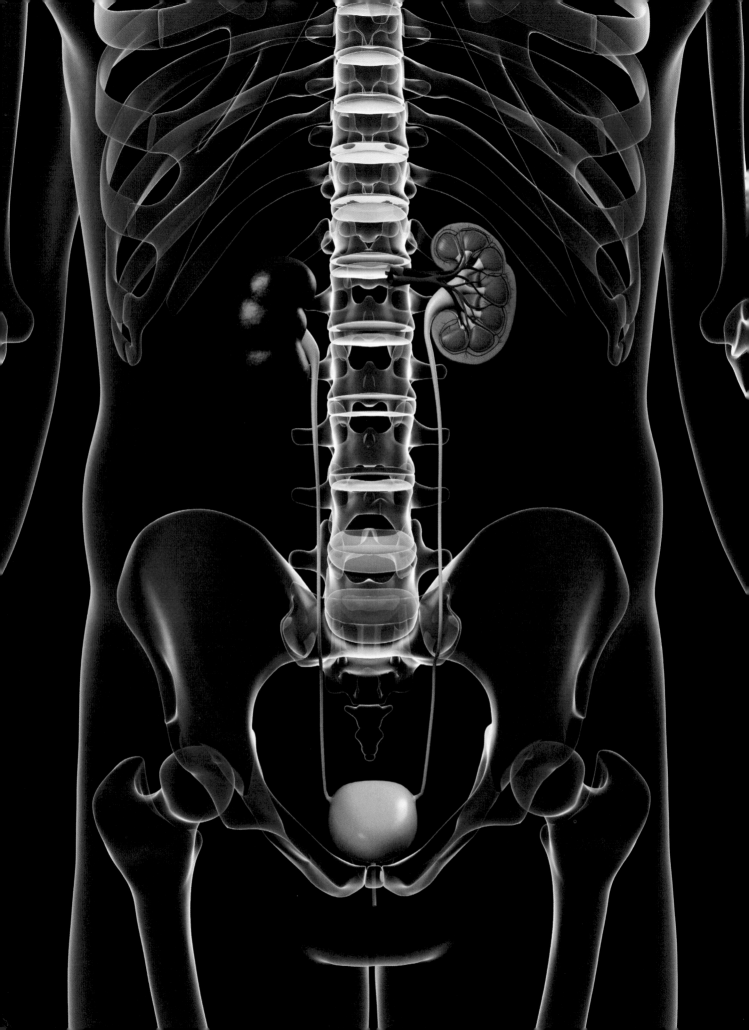

Acute kidney injury and chronic kidney disease

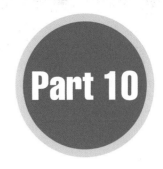

Part 10

Chapters

Don't forget to visit the companion website for this book
www.ataglanceseries.com/renalsystem

41 Acute kidney injury: pathophysiology 100
42 Acute kidney injury: clinical aspects 102
43 Chronic kidney disease and kidney function in the elderly 104
44 Severe chronic kidney disease and renal bone disease 106
45 Severe chronic kidney disease: clinical complications and their management 108
46 Treatment of kidney failure with dialysis 110
47 Peritoneal dialysis and continuous hemofiltration 112
48 Renal transplantation 114
49 Global kidney medicine 116

41 Acute kidney injury: pathophysiology

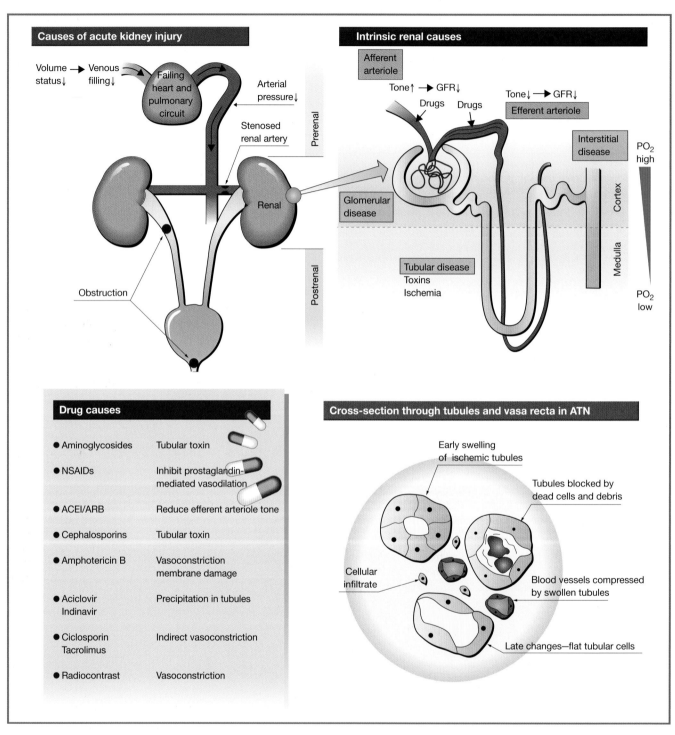

Causes of acute kidney injury

Volume status↓ → Venous filling↓ → Failing heart and pulmonary circuit

Arterial pressure↓

Stenosed renal artery

Renal

Obstruction

Prerenal

Postrenal

Intrinsic renal causes

Afferent arteriole

Tone↑ → GFR↓

Drugs   Drugs

Tone↓ → GFR↓

Efferent arteriole

Glomerular disease

Interstitial disease

Cortex

Medulla

PO₂ high

PO₂ low

Tubular disease
Toxins
Ischemia

Drug causes

- Aminoglycosides — Tubular toxin
- NSAIDs — Inhibit prostaglandin-mediated vasodilation
- ACEI/ARB — Reduce efferent arteriole tone
- Cephalosporins — Tubular toxin
- Amphotericin B — Vasoconstriction membrane damage
- Aciclovir Indinavir — Precipitation in tubules
- Ciclosporin Tacrolimus — Indirect vasoconstriction
- Radiocontrast — Vasoconstriction

Cross-section through tubules and vasa recta in ATN

Early swelling of ischemic tubules

Tubules blocked by dead cells and debris

Cellular infiltrate

Blood vessels compressed by swollen tubules

Late changes—flat tubular cells

The Renal System at a Glance, Fourth Edition. Chris O'Callaghan. © 2017 John Wiley & Sons, Ltd. Published 2017 by John Wiley & Sons, Ltd.
Companion website: www.ataglanceseries.com/renalsystem

Acute kidney injury (AKI) arises when there is an acute fall in glomerular filtration rate (GFR) and substances that are usually excreted by the kidneys accumulate in the blood. AKI can be caused by inadequate renal perfusion (prerenal), intrinsic renal disease (renal), and urinary tract obstruction (postrenal). Prerenal conditions account for 50–65% of cases, postrenal for 15%, and renal for the remaining 20–35%. In developing countries, obstetric complications and infections such as malaria are important causes (Chapter 49). The overall mortality rate is around 30–70%, depending on age and the presence of other organ failure or disease. Of survivors, 60% regain normal renal function, but 15–30% have renal impairment, and around 5–10% develop end-stage renal disease.

Prerenal disease

Inadequate cardiac function, circulatory volume depletion, and obstruction of the arterial supply to the kidneys can all impair renal perfusion. The resulting renal ischemia can cause acute tubular necrosis (ATN).

Postrenal disease

Obstruction to urine flow causes back-pressure which inhibits filtration. The subsequent swelling compresses blood vessels, causing ischemia. AKI arises only if both kidneys are obstructed or if there is only one functioning kidney and that kidney is obstructed. The cause of the obstruction can be within the urinary tract (such as a stone), within the wall of the tract (such as a tumor or stricture), or outside the wall (such as compression by a mass or fibrotic process).

Intrinsic renal disease

Intrinsic renal causes of AKI are glomerular disease, tubulointerstitial disease, and drugs or toxins. The main glomerular causes of AKI are acute or rapidly progressive glomerulonephritis, Goodpasture's syndrome, vasculitis, and proliferative glomerulonephritis associated with a multisystem disease or infection.

Tubular toxins

Tubular injury can result from ischemia, or from toxic effects of exogenous compounds such as drugs, heavy metals, and contrast media or endogenous compounds such as hemoglobin or myoglobin. Exercise, trauma, or other causes of muscle damage cause rhabdomyolysis with myoglobin release. Hemolysis destroys red cells, releasing hemoglobin. Hemolytic uremic syndrome consists of hemolysis and AKI and can follow infection with *Escherichia coli* serotype O157:H7. Both hemoglobin and myoglobin are filtered in the glomerulus and are toxic to tubular cells. Acute hypercalcemia can cause AKI not only by renal vasoconstriction, but also by calcium phosphate precipitation in the tubules. In myeloma, light chain precipitation in the tubules can cause cast nephropathy and AKI (see Chapter 34). Crystals forming in the tubules can cause tubular injury and obstruction (e.g., gout, aciclovir, or indinavir crystals).

Drugs

Any drug can cause an allergic tubulointerstitial nephritis, especially nonsteroidal anti-inflammatory drugs (NSAIDs), diuretics, proton pump inhibitors, and antibiotics (see Chapter 36). Some drugs cause AKI through other mechanisms (see figure). **Aminoglycoside** antibiotics are tubular toxins which cause acute tubular necrosis.

NSAIDs and vessel tone

Normally, there is a tonic prostaglandin-induced vasodilation of renal arterioles. NSAIDs inhibit prostaglandin synthesis. This leads to vasoconstriction, which reduces renal blood flow. If there is volume depletion, the vasoconstrictive drive may be very strong, causing a serious fall in the GFR. Risk factors for NSAID-induced kidney injury are volume depletion, diuretic use, pre-existing renal impairment, and an edema state (congestive heart failure, liver cirrhosis, or nephrotic syndrome). In renal artery stenosis (see Chapter 8), angiotensin II causes efferent arteriolar constriction to maintain the GFR. **ACE inhibitors or angiotensin II receptor blockers** can block this constriction, causing a large fall in the GFR.

Pathophysiology of acute tubular necrosis

Most AKI results from acute tubular necrosis. This usually arises when there is renal hypoperfusion, with renal ischemia, in combination with other factors such as sepsis or circulating tubular toxins or nephrotoxic drugs. Acute tubular necrosis is associated with tubular cell death and shedding into the tubular lumen, resulting in tubular blockage (see Chapter 36). This raises the tubular pressure, which eventually stops further glomerular filtration. Swollen tubules also compress the nearby vasa recta, which further reduces perfusion.

Vascular effects of ischemia

Various factors can exacerbate ischemia, including disordered regulation of vascular tone after an initial ischemic insult. Ischemic renal endothelium releases the vasoconstrictor endothelin; as well as increased levels of vasoconstrictors, including angiotensin II, catecholamines, and arachidonic acid metabolites, there may be low levels of locally acting vasodilators such as prostacyclin (PGI2) and nitric oxide (NO). Initially, tubular damage reduces sodium reabsorption. This increases tubular sodium concentrations at the macula densa, stimulating tubuloglomerular feedback, causing further vasoconstriction due to the release of adenosine (see Chapter 6).

Cellular mechanisms of tubular damage

A number of mechanisms are implicated in the process of tubular injury. Ischemia causes production of oxygen free radicals. These damage cellular and mitochondrial membrane lipids and can lead to cell death. Ischemia depletes ATP and so inhibits energy-dependent calcium efflux from cells. Elevated intracellular calcium levels interfere with metabolic processes. Ischemic cells can lose their actin cytoskeletal integrity and detach from the basement membrane. Ischemic cells can also lose their membrane polarity, allowing channels to move around the membrane, which disrupts tubular transport function. Apoptosis and necrosis of tubular cells are common.

42 Acute kidney injury: clinical aspects

Key features to assess in AKI

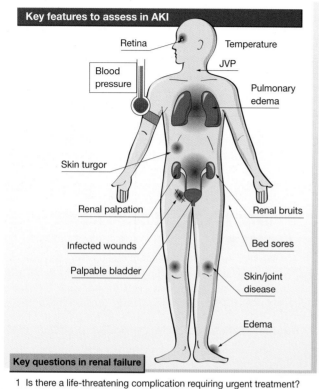

Retina
Temperature
JVP
Blood pressure
Pulmonary edema
Skin turgor
Renal palpation
Renal bruits
Infected wounds
Bed sores
Palpable bladder
Skin/joint disease
Edema

Key questions in renal failure

1 Is there a life-threatening complication requiring urgent treatment?
2 Is the renal failure acute or chronic?
3 If acute, is it prerenal, renal, or postrenal?
   – if pre- or postrenal, treat cause
4 If it is renal, what is the diagnosis?

Common features in AKI in hospital

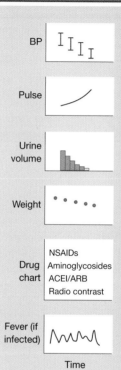

BP
Pulse
Urine volume
Weight
Drug chart
  NSAIDs
  Aminoglycosides
  ACEI/ARB
  Radio contrast
Fever (if infected)
Time

General pattern of acute kidney injury

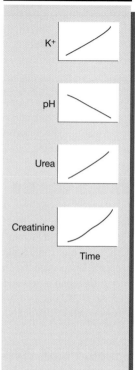

K+
pH
Urea
Creatinine
Time

Renal causes of AKI

Diagnosis	Clinical features	Investigations
Rhabdomyolysis	Muscle pain	CK↑, myoglobinuria
Glomerulonephritis		Red cell casts
● Goodpasture's diseas	Pulmonary hemorrhage	Anti-GBM antibodies↑
● Vasculitis	±Systemic features, sinusitis, rash,	ANCA↑ (anti neutrophil cytoplasmic antibodies)
● SLE	joint/neurological signs, rash	Anti-dsDNA↑, anti nuclear antibodies
Interstitial nephritis	Drug cause	Eosinophils↑, (blood and urine), Hb↓, hemolysis
Hemolytic uremic syndrome	Diarrhea	Granular tubular casts
Acute tubular necrosis	Multiple factors, especially in hospitals	

Most acute kidney injury arises in hospital from fluid depletion, sepsis, or drug toxicity, especially after surgery, trauma, or burns. There is usually a fall in urine output and a rise in serum urea and creatinine. A urine output of less than 400 mL/day is termed oliguria. It is important to identify people at risk of AKI and take steps to prevent AKI wherever possible.

History

A history may indicate pre-existing renal impairment, hypertension, or diabetes mellitus, which all predispose to renal ischemia. Frank hematuria followed by oliguria suggests glomerulonephritis; hemoptysis suggests Goodpasture's syndrome; a recent throat or skin infection suggests post-infectious glomerulonephritis. In men, urinary frequency, nocturia, and a poor stream with hesitancy and dribbling suggest postrenal obstruction resulting from prostate disease. Muscle pain and swelling after exercise suggest rhabdomyolysis. Recent gastroenteritis can indicate *Escherichia coli*-associated hemolytic uremic syndrome. The **past medical history** may reveal an underlying multisystem disease associated with glomerulonephritis, vascular disease (associated with renal artery stenosis), malignancy (associated with hypercalcemia), or chronic infection such as osteomyelitis or abnormal heart valves

The Renal System at a Glance, Fourth Edition. Chris O'Callaghan. © 2017 John Wiley & Sons, Ltd. Published 2017 by John Wiley & Sons, Ltd.
Companion website: www.ataglanceseries.com/renalsystem

that are vulnerable to endocarditis. The **drug history** should include possible self-poisoning and analgesic use. Chronic kidney disease (Chapter 43) is a risk factor for AKI.

Examination

Assess the fluid volume status. Look for signs of a multisystem disease, of cholesterol emboli, and of intravenous drug use. Muscle swelling or tenderness suggests rhabdomyolysis. The eyes may have hypertensive, diabetic, or other diagnostic changes. Examine all bedsores, and surgical and traumatic wounds for sepsis. Pulse, blood pressure (lying and standing if necessary), jugular venous pressure, and a cardiac examination may indicate volume depletion, cardiac lesions, or pericarditis. Examine the chest for pulmonary edema and evidence of infection or bleeding. Upper airway disease or sinusitis suggests granulomatosis with polyangiitis (GPA, Wegener's disease). Polycystic kidneys may be palpable and a large palpable bladder suggests obstruction. Rectal examination may demonstrate prostate or pelvic disease.

Investigations

Blood biochemistry

Hyperkalemia and severe acidosis can cause cardiac arrest. In rhabdomyolysis, creatine kinase is released from muscle and plasma creatinine kinase levels are high.

Hematology

Anemia can result from blood loss, suppressed erythropoiesis, low erythropoietin levels, or hemolysis. A high eosinophil count suggests acute interstitial nephritis. Hemolytic uremic syndrome causes hemolysis with anemia, damaged red blood cells, and a low platelet count.

Urine

Urine dipstick, microscopy, and culture should be performed. Leucocytes and nitrites indicate infection. Heavy proteinuria suggests glomerulonephritis or myeloma. Hematuria indicates renal or postrenal disease, but can be caused by urinary catheterization. Myoglobin in the urine suggests rhabdomyolysis, and hemoglobin in the urine suggests hemolysis. Granular tubular casts may occur in acute tubular necrosis. Red cell casts are diagnostic of glomerular disease. Eosinophils in the urine suggest interstitial nephritis.

Radiology

Ultrasonography is mandatory to exclude obstruction if no cause for the AKI has been identified and will also determine the size of the kidneys. Small kidneys indicate chronic kidney disease. Angiography or ultrasonographic Doppler studies or radioisotopic methods can evaluate renal perfusion.

Immunology

Complement levels are low in systemic lupus erythematosus and post-infectious glomerulonephritis. Antiglomerular basement membrane antibodies suggest Goodpasture's syndrome, and antineutrophil cytoplasmic antibodies (ANCAs) suggest vasculitis. Antinuclear antibodies or antibodies to double-stranded DNA suggest systemic lupus erythematosus. Myeloma may be indicated by the presence of antibody free light chains (Bence Jones protein) in the urine or a monoclonal band in plasma (see Chapter 34).

Microbiology and histology

Cultures should be taken to exclude sepsis and, if the etiology of renal disease is unclear, a renal biopsy should be performed.

Diagnosis

The KDIGO (Kidney Disease: Improving Global Outcome) classification of AKI has three stages which takes into account the extent of the rise in creatinine (or fall in eGFR) and of the fall in urine output. Both KDIGO and NICE (UK National Institute for Health and Care Excellence) recommends diagnosing AKI if one of the following is present: a rise in creatinine of ≥ 26 µmol/L within 48 h, a rise of $\geq 50\%$ in creatinine or fall of $\geq 25\%$ in eGFR within 7 days, urine output <0.5 mL/kg/h for >6 h.

Management

Prerenal or postrenal causes must be corrected urgently. Intrinsic renal disease is treated according to its type. Regardless of the etiology, certain basic measures are routine.

Electrolytes

Plasma electrolytes should be measured daily. Potassium intake should be restricted and diuretics or renal replacement therapy used to prevent hyperkalemia.

Acid

Acid inhibits metabolic processes. Severe acidosis with inadequate renal function must be treated with renal replacement therapy.

Volume

Regularly assess the body fluid volume. When necessary, measure the central venous pressure with an internal jugular or subclavian venous catheter. Monitor the fluid intake and urine and other fluid output. Urinary catheterization provides accurate urine volumes, but is an infection risk. Daily insensible losses vary with a minimum of 500 mL and around 500 mL extra per °C of fever. Daily weighing of patients can guide volume replacement. Volume replacement should match known and insensible losses.

Pulmonary edema

The patient should be sat up and given oxygen. Diuretics are given if there is any renal function. If not, renal replacement therapy must be instituted urgently. In the meantime, nitrates and opiates provide vasodilation. If necessary, venesect 200–500 mL blood and ventilate the patient with positive end-expiratory pressures.

General measures

Correct any hypoxia with oxygen and, if necessary, ventilation. Cardiac output should be maintained with inotropes. Hemoglobin should be kept above 10 g/dL to maintain tissue oxygenation. Patients are often hypercatabolic and must be fed nasogastrically or parenterally if they cannot eat. Hypertension should be controlled by adjusting fluid balance and antihypertensives if necessary.

Renal replacement therapy

Absolute indications for renal replacement therapy include hyperkalemia, acidosis, pulmonary edema, and severe uremic complications. Hemodialysis can be poorly tolerated by hemodynamically unstable patients. Continuous hemofiltration, which is slower, is usually better tolerated.

43 Chronic kidney disease and kidney function in the elderly

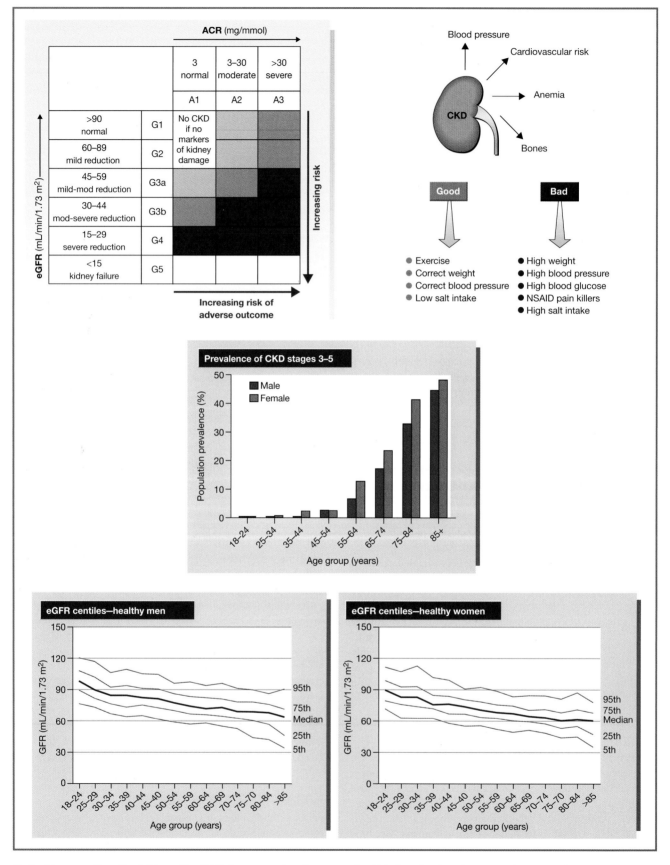

		ACR (mg/mmol)		
		3 normal	3–30 moderate	>30 severe
		A1	A2	A3
>90 normal	G1	No CKD if no markers of kidney damage		
60–89 mild reduction	G2			
45–59 mild-mod reduction	G3a			
30–44 mod-severe reduction	G3b			
15–29 severe reduction	G4			
<15 kidney failure	G5			

eGFR (mL/min/1.73 m²)

Increasing risk

Increasing risk of adverse outcome

CKD → Blood pressure, Cardiovascular risk, Anemia, Bones

Good
- Exercise
- Correct weight
- Correct blood pressure
- Low salt intake

Bad
- High weight
- High blood pressure
- High blood glucose
- NSAID pain killers
- High salt intake

Prevalence of CKD stages 3–5

Male / Female

Population prevalence (%) — Age group (years): 18–24, 25–34, 35–44, 45–54, 55–64, 65–74, 75–84, 85+

eGFR centiles—healthy men

GFR (mL/min/1.73 m²) — Age group (years): 18–24, 25–29, 30–34, 35–39, 40–44, 45–40, 50–54, 55–59, 60–64, 65–69, 70–74, 75–70, 80–84, >85

95th, 75th, Median, 25th, 5th

eGFR centiles—healthy women

GFR (mL/min/1.73 m²) — Age group (years): 18–24, 25–29, 30–34, 35–39, 40–44, 45–40, 50–54, 55–59, 60–64, 65–69, 70–74, 75–70, 80–84, >85

95th, 75th, Median, 25th, 5th

The Renal System at a Glance, Fourth Edition. Chris O'Callaghan. © 2017 John Wiley & Sons, Ltd. Published 2017 by John Wiley & Sons, Ltd.
Companion website: www.ataglanceseries.com/renalsystem

Chronic kidney disease (CKD) is reduced kidney function or kidney disease of any form that has been present for some time. CKD is common throughout the world, with an estimated prevalence of 5–15% in some countries. The prevalence is increasing because people are living longer than they used to and because of an increase in obesity and Type 2 diabetes mellitus, both of which can cause kidney damage. CKD is important for several reasons. First, it is associated with an increased risk of vascular disease such as heart attacks and strokes. Second, in some patients it will progress, causing complications and requiring renal replacement therapy (see Chapters 44–48). Third, it affects which drugs may be safely prescribed to the patient. In people of black African ethnicity, variants in the APOL1 gene are associated with a higher prevalence of CKD.

Changes in kidney function with age

Kidney function declines with age in all people, and the prevalence of diabetes mellitus and hypertension, which can cause renal impairment, increases with age. Therefore, as the number of older people in the population increases, so does the number of people with impaired renal function. It is unclear whether it is inevitable that renal function declines with age or whether this decline results from our lifestyle. Nevertheless, with our current lifestyles, renal function deteriorates substantially with age, even in the absence of any specific renal disease, and we cannot completely prevent this. This means that many old people will have a low glomerular filtration rate (GFR), but will not have a specific kidney condition. For this reason, aggressive investigation of renal impairment in elderly people is only likely to be useful if their renal function is outside the normal range for their age group.

The use of the term "kidney disease" has been questioned for older patients with a low estimated GFR (eGFR), but no specific kidney disease. However, renal impairment in the elderly cannot be dismissed because it has significant consequences. For example, drugs that are excreted by the kidneys will accumulate and must be used with caution in elderly people with relatively poor renal function. Similarly, nonsteroidal anti-inflammatory drugs reduce GFR, and in elderly patients who already have a low GFR, these drugs can reduce renal function to dangerous levels.

eGFR reporting

As discussed in Chapter 5, blood creatinine levels do not rise significantly until there is a large fall in GFR, but GFR is difficult to measure accurately. Estimates of GFR based on creatinine clearance are not very reliable, partly because patients have to remember to collect all their urine in a 24-h period. It is possible to estimate GFR from serum creatinine and other information such as age and gender. Most national guidelines recommend the use of the CKD-EPI formula to calculate this eGFR. As with true GFR, eGFR falls with age, so that older patients will be expected

to have a lower eGFR than younger patients. Men typically have higher eGFRs than women. People of black African ethnicity have higher plasma creatinine levels than white people with equivalent renal function, so their eGFR should be increased by about 20% if their ethnicity has not already been taken into account. The eGFR is much less accurate with relatively good kidney function and should be interpreted with caution when the eGFR is predicted to be >60 mL/min. Blood cystatin C levels can be used to estimate GFR and these estimates correlate better with measured GFR than creatinine-based eGFRs. This can be useful in those with creatinine-based eGFRs of 45–59 mL/min/1.73 m^2 but no other indications of CKD. CKD has been divided into stages according to the eGFR and the level of albuminuria.

Assessment of chronic kidney disease

Most patients with CKD are asymptomatic and are usually identified by blood tests taken for another reason. Clinical assessment has two goals: first, to determine whether there is a specific cause for the kidney disease that might be treatable; second, to assess the severity of the kidney disease to determine what general measures need to be taken, such as blood pressure control.

The history and examination may identify specific causes of renal impairment, such as a large bladder indicating urinary obstruction. Blood pressure must be carefully assessed. Urine should be analyzed for blood and protein. At low levels of proteinuria, it is helpful to assess the urine albumin : creatinine ratio (ACR). Other investigations may be appropriate depending on the clinical context, in particular, ultrasound scanning of the kidneys to examine the anatomy and exclude obstruction, especially in older men who may have enlarged prostate glands.

Management of chronic kidney disease

If there is a specific treatable cause of kidney disease, then this should be treated. For most patients, this is not the case and management consists mainly of good blood pressure control, which can slow the rate of renal deterioration. In patients with significant proteinuria, stricter targets are set for blood pressure control. In all patients with CKD, kidney function must be monitored, and if severe CKD develops, appropriate treatments can be put in place (see Chapters 44–48). Patients with CKD have an increased risk of acute kidney injury (Chapter 42). Patients with CKD are at risk of vascular disease, so other measures that reduce their risk of vascular disease are sensible, such as avoiding smoking and lowering lipid levels. Lifestyle changes that help to lower blood pressure are beneficial, such as weight control, increased exercise, reduced salt intake, reduced alcohol intake, and reduced dietary salt intake. Drugs such as nonsteroidal anti-inflammatory drugs that have undesirable renal effects should be avoided.

Severe chronic kidney disease and renal bone disease

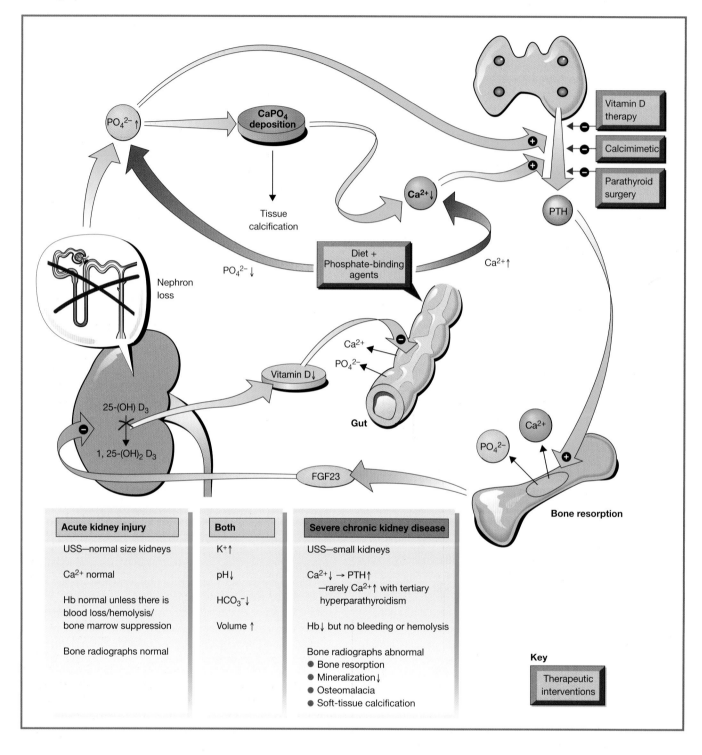

Acute kidney injury	Both	Severe chronic kidney disease
USS—normal size kidneys	$K^+\uparrow$	USS—small kidneys
Ca^{2+} normal	$pH\downarrow$	$Ca^{2+}\downarrow \rightarrow PTH\uparrow$ —rarely $Ca^{2+}\uparrow$ with tertiary hyperparathyroidism
Hb normal unless there is blood loss/hemolysis/ bone marrow suppression	$HCO_3^-\downarrow$	Hb$\downarrow$ but no bleeding or hemolysis
Bone radiographs normal	Volume $\uparrow$	Bone radiographs abnormal • Bone resorption • Mineralization$\downarrow$ • Osteomalacia • Soft-tissue calcification

Key

Therapeutic interventions

The Renal System at a Glance, Fourth Edition. Chris O'Callaghan. © 2017 John Wiley & Sons, Ltd. Published 2017 by John Wiley & Sons, Ltd.
Companion website: www.ataglanceseries.com/renalsystem

Severe chronic kidney disease with severe loss of renal function is often referred to as chronic renal failure. Any disease process causing progressive nephron loss can cause chronic kidney disease. As the number of functioning nephrons declines, the surviving nephrons compensate by increasing filtration and solute reabsorption. Unfortunately, this damages the remaining nephrons and accelerates nephron loss. *End-stage renal disease* occurs when patients require renal replacement therapy with dialysis or transplantation.

Complications of severe chronic kidney disease are caused by the accumulation of substances that are normally excreted by the kidney, and by inadequate production of vitamin D and erythropoietin by the kidney. The *uremic syndrome* refers to the complications of chronic renal failure such as anemia, confusion, coma, asterixis, seizures, pericardial effusion, itch, and bone disease. Renal replacement therapy improves these problems, but patients with end-stage renal disease have a higher morbidity and mortality than the rest of the population.

Distinction between acute kidney injury and severe chronic kidney disease

Severe acute kidney injury and chronic kidney disease both raise plasma potassium, urea, and creatinine, and cause metabolic acidosis. In severe chronic kidney disease, there is usually evidence of chronic complications, including anemia caused by inadequate erythropoietin, and bone disease, typically with a low calcium, a raised phosphate, and a high parathyroid hormone (PTH) level. Plasma calcium is characteristically low in severe chronic kidney disease, unless tertiary hyperparathyroidism is present (see Chapter 27). The key finding in severe chronic kidney disease is small kidneys on ultrasonography (USS). The reduction in size is caused by atrophy and fibrosis.

Acute problems in chronic kidney disease

Acute problems can occur in both acute and chronic renal failure. Emergency treatment with dialysis or hemofiltration may be needed for life-threatening hyperkalemia, severe acidosis, pulmonary edema, and uremic symptoms. Sudden deterioration in patients with renal impairment who are not yet on dialysis can be triggered by severe hypertension, urinary tract infection, or nephrotoxic drugs. Nonsteroidal anti-inflammatory drugs or angiotensin-converting enzyme inhibitors can cause renal deterioration by adversely affecting glomerular blood flow.

Renal bone disease and calcium and phosphate metabolism

Renal bone disease can cause bone pain, especially in the lower back, hips, and legs, and is often associated with proximal myopathy and soft tissue calcification. Bone alkaline phosphatase is usually elevated. Two types of renal bone disease can be distinguished by bone biopsy. Most renal bone disease is conventional or **high-turnover bone disease**, in which there

is excess PTH. The PTH stimulates bone resorption, and the new bone that replaces it has disordered collagen. Radiographs may show subperiosteal resorption in the phalanges, erosion of the phalangeal tufts, and erosion of the clavicle heads. In **low-turnover bone disease**, PTH levels are low. Bone turnover is low and there is osteomalacia with poorly mineralized bone. This bone disease arises if calcium intake and plasma calcium levels are high enough to suppress PTH secretion below the level required for healthy bone turnover. Vitamin D levels may also be low. Radiographs may show multiple fractures or pseudofractures (radiolucent cortical zones perpendicular to the bone surface).

Causes of high-turnover renal bone disease

The main causes of renal bone disease are renal phosphate retention and inadequate renal vitamin D production. Vitamin D deficiency reduces gut calcium and phosphate absorption but, with renal phosphate retention, the net result is a rise in phosphate and a fall in calcium. The rise in phosphate further lowers the calcium by causing calcium phosphate deposition in tissues. The hypocalcemia stimulates a rise in PTH, causing secondary hyperparathyroidism (see Chapter 27). Eventually, PTH secretion can become autonomous and fails to fall even if calcium rises as a result of bone mobilization. This is termed tertiary hyperparathyroidism. Other factors can exacerbate renal bone disease. A high phosphate level directly stimulates PTH secretion and directly inhibits renal vitamin D production. Normally, vitamin D binds to receptors on parathyroid cells and inhibits PTH secretion, so vitamin D deficiency causes excess PTH secretion. Acidosis stimulates bone resorption. FGF23 levels are elevated in late CKD and this further inhibits renal vitamin D production (Chapter 26). Renal klotho production falls in CKD and klotho deficiency may contribute to the tissue and vascular calcification which can arise with late CKD.

Treatment of high-turnover renal bone disease

Dialysis removes some phosphate from the plasma. However, for good phosphate control, dietary phosphate intake must be reduced and phosphate-binding compounds taken with food. Compounds, containing calcium or lanthanum or synthetic resins, bind dietary phosphate, blocking its absorption in the gut. Vitamin D given as 1,25-dihydroxy-vitamin D_3 [1,25-$(OH)_2$-D_3 or calcitriol] or 1-hydroxy-vitamin D_3 [1-(OH)-D_3 or alfacalcidol] inhibits PTH secretion and bone turnover, and raises plasma calcium by increasing dietary calcium absorption. It may also help bone pain and proximal myopathy. Treatment should reduce PTH levels sufficiently to prevent high-turnover bone disease without causing a dynamic low-turnover bone disease. If PTH does not fall when calcium levels rise and vitamin D is administered, calcimimetic drugs, such as cinacalcet, which reduce PTH levels (see Chapter 27), or surgical removal of parathyroid gland tissue, are usually required. Bone disease may improve with rigorous correction of acidosis by dialysis and if necessary, oral calcium carbonate or sodium bicarbonate.

45 Severe chronic kidney disease: clinical complications and their management

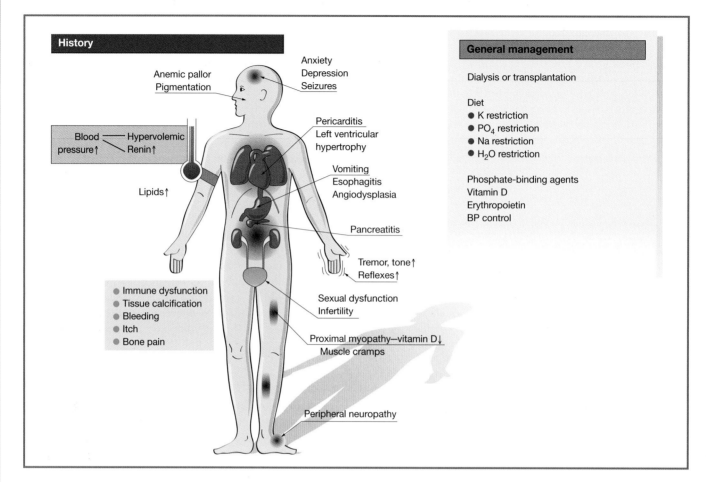

History

Anemic pallor
Pigmentation

Anxiety
Depression
Seizures

Blood pressure↑ — Hypervolemic
— Renin↑

Pericarditis
Left ventricular hypertrophy

Lipids↑

Vomiting
Esophagitis
Angiodysplasia

Pancreatitis

Tremor, tone↑
Reflexes↑

● Immune dysfunction
● Tissue calcification
● Bleeding
● Itch
● Bone pain

Sexual dysfunction
Infertility

Proximal myopathy—vitamin D↓
Muscle cramps

Peripheral neuropathy

General management

Dialysis or transplantation

Diet
● K restriction
● PO$_4$ restriction
● Na restriction
● H$_2$O restriction

Phosphate-binding agents
Vitamin D
Erythropoietin
BP control

Many complications arise as renal function declines. Renal bone disease is considered in Chapter 44.

Hematological complications

Anemia in chronic kidney disease is caused by inadequate erythropoietin production by the kidney (see Chapter 9) and is treated by giving erythropoietin subcutaneously or intravenously. This works only if iron, folate, and vitamin B$_{12}$ levels are adequate and the patient is otherwise well. Very rarely antibodies can develop against administered erythropoietin resulting in aplastic anemia. In CKD, hepcidin production from the liver is increased and this reduces iron availability for red cell formation (Chapter 9)

Although laboratory clotting times are normal, platelet function is impaired and the **bleeding time** (the time for bleeding from a cut to stop) is increased. The bleeding time can be improved by efficient dialysis, correction of anemia with

erythropoietin, and administration of conjugated estrogens. Synthetic vasopressin (desmopressin or DDAVP) increases von Willebrand's factor levels and transiently reduces the bleeding time.

Vascular disease and hypertension

Vascular disease is the major cause of death in severe chronic kidney disease. In patients who do not have diabetes, hypertension is an important risk factor, but vascular calcification also plays a role (Chapter 44). Much hypertension in severe chronic kidney disease results from hypervolemia caused by sodium and water retention. This is not usually severe enough to cause edema, but there may be a triple cardiac rhythm. Such hypertension usually responds to sodium restriction, and control of body volume with dialysis. If renal function is sufficient, furosemide can be useful.

Hypertension that does not respond to a reduction in body volume is often associated with excess renin production. Excess sympathetic activity may also contribute. Vasoconstrictors such

The Renal System at a Glance, Fourth Edition. Chris O'Callaghan. © 2017 John Wiley & Sons, Ltd. Published 2017 by John Wiley & Sons, Ltd.
Companion website: www.ataglanceseries.com/renalsystem

as endothelin, antidiuretic hormone (ADH or vasopressin), norepinephrine (noradrenaline), or a deficiency of the vasodilator nitric oxide might also play a role in this hypertension. If blood pressure cannot be controlled with angiotensin-converting enzyme inhibitors, angiotensin receptor blockers, vasodilators, or β-blockers, nephrectomy is sometimes helpful. However, renal artery stenosis should be excluded as a cause of the hypertension because it is often treatable by balloon angioplasty.

Dehydration

A loss of renal function usually causes sodium and water retention as a result of nephron loss. However, some patients maintain some filtration, but lose tubular function, and therefore excrete very dilute urine, which can lead to dehydration.

Skin

Itch is the most common skin complaint. It often arises with secondary or tertiary hyperparathyroidism and may result from calcium phosphate deposition in the tissues. Itch can be helped by the control of phosphate levels and by creams that prevent dry skin. Uremic frost is the precipitation of urea crystals on the skin and occurs only in severe uremia. Skin pigmentation can occur and anemia can cause pallor.

Gastrointestinal

Although gastrin levels are elevated, peptic ulceration is no more common in patients with chronic kidney disease than in the general population. However, symptoms of nausea, vomiting, anorexia, and heartburn are common, and there is a higher incidence of esophagitis and angiodysplasia, both of which can lead to bleeding. There is also a higher incidence of pancreatitis. Taste disturbance may be associated with a urine-like smell to the breath.

Endocrine

In men, severe chronic kidney disease can cause loss of libido, impotence, and low sperm count and motility. In women, there is often loss of libido, reduced ovulation, and infertility. Abnormal growth hormone cycles contribute to growth retardation in children and loss of muscle mass in adults.

Neurological and psychiatric

Untreated end-stage renal disease can cause fatigue, diminished consciousness, and even coma, often with signs of neurological irritation (including tremor, asterixis, agitation, meningism, increased muscle tone with myoclonus, ankle clonus, hyperreflexia, extensor plantars, and ultimately, seizures). Na^+/K^+ ATPase activity is impaired in uremia and there are parathyroid hormone (PTH)-dependent changes in membrane calcium transport, which may contribute to abnormal neurotransmission.

Peripheral neuropathies can occur. The typical presentation is of a distal sensorimotor neuropathy, with glove and stocking sensory loss and distal muscle weakness and wasting. This is usually symmetrical, but can be an isolated mononeuropathy and can affect the cranial nerves. Autonomic neuropathy can also occur. Myopathy can be caused by vitamin D deficiency, hypocalcemia, hypophosphatemia, and excess PTH. Sleep disorder is common. Restless legs or muscle cramps also occur and sometimes respond to quinine sulfate. Psychiatric disturbances including depression and anxiety are common and there is an increased risk of suicide.

Immunological

Immunological function is impaired in severe chronic kidney disease and infection is common. Uremia suppresses the function of most immune cells, and dialysis itself can inappropriately activate immune effectors, such as complement.

Lipids

Hyperlipidemia is common, especially hypertriglyceridemia resulting from decreased triglyceride catabolism. Lipid levels are higher in patients on peritoneal dialysis than in those on hemodialysis, probably as a result of the loss of regulatory plasma proteins such as apolipoprotein A-1 across the peritoneal membranes. Statins are usually given to lower cholesterol levels.

Cardiac disease

Pericarditis can occur and is more likely if urea or phosphate levels are high or there is severe secondary hyperparathyroidism. Fluid overload and hypertension can cause left ventricular hypertrophy or a dilated cardiomyopathy. A large arteriovenous dialysis fistula can use up a considerable proportion of cardiac output, reducing the available cardiac output for the rest of the body.

Conservative management of severe chronic kidney disease

Management involves dietary restriction of potassium, phosphate, sodium, and water intake to avoid hyperkalemia, bone disease, and hypervolemia. Mild sustained hypervolemia can cause hypertension, leading to vascular disease and left ventricular hypertrophy. Severe hypervolemia causes pulmonary edema. Blood pressure that cannot be controlled by strict fluid balance should be treated with angiotensin-converting enzyme inhibitors, angiotensin receptor blockers, β-blockers, or vasodilators. Anemia should be treated with erythropoietin, after ensuring that there is no gastrointestinal or excessive menstrual blood loss and that iron, folate, and vitamin B_{12} levels are adequate. Intravenous iron therapy may be required. Bone disease is treated by reducing phosphate intake, taking phosphate-binding compounds with meals, and taking vitamin D as either 1-hydroxy-vitamin D_3 or 1,25-dihydroxy-vitamin D_3. Hyperparathyroidism may be treated with cinacalcet or parathyroidectomy. When chronic kidney disease is severe, dialysis or renal transplantation is usually required in addition to these measures. The quality of life of patients who decline these options can be improved by management of the complications of severe chronic kidney disease, especially anemia. In elderly patients the morbidity of dialysis can be high and it may not increase survival in frail elderly patients.

46 Treatment of kidney failure with dialysis

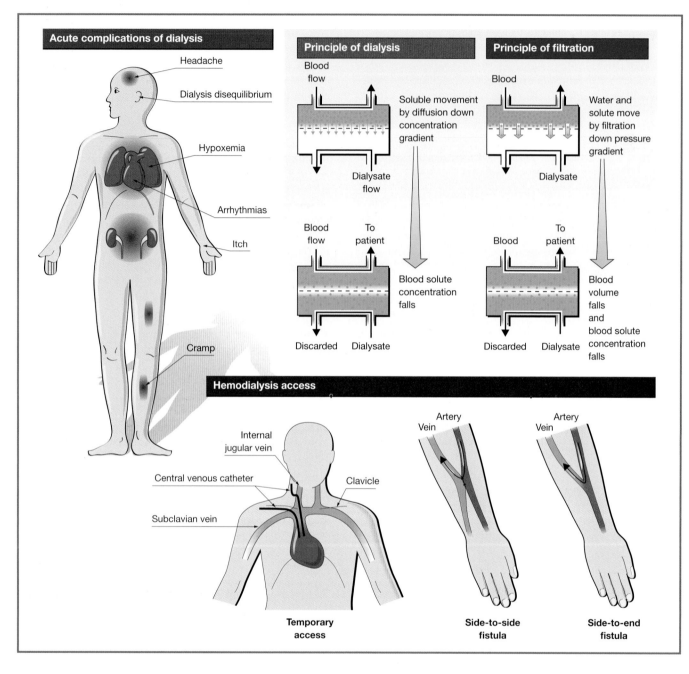

Acute complications of dialysis

Headache

Dialysis disequilibrium

Hypoxemia

Arrhythmias

Itch

Cramp

Principle of dialysis

Blood flow

Dialysate flow

Soluble movement by diffusion down concentration gradient

Blood flow — To patient

Discarded — Dialysate

Blood solute concentration falls

Principle of filtration

Blood

Dialysate

Water and solute move by filtration down pressure gradient

Blood — To patient

Discarded — Dialysate

Blood volume falls and blood solute concentration falls

Hemodialysis access

Internal jugular vein

Central venous catheter

Clavicle

Subclavian vein

Temporary access

Artery / Vein

Side-to-side fistula

Artery / Vein

Side-to-end fistula

End-stage renal disease results from progressive chronic kidney disease or unrecovered acute kidney injury. Without renal replacement therapy, death from metabolic derangement follows rapidly. Transplantation is the best treatment, but because there is a shortage of organs, patients usually start dialysis while waiting for a transplant. Dialysis is started to treat or to prevent life-threatening hyperkalemia, acidosis, or hypervolemic pulmonary edema, or to treat complications of chronic renal failure such as pericarditis, neuropathy, seizures, and coma.

The number of patients on renal replacement therapy has progressively risen since dialysis began, because older and sicker patients can now be safely dialyzed.

Hemodialysis

Modern renal replacement uses **dialysis** to remove unwanted solutes by diffusion and **hemofiltration** to remove water, which carries with it unwanted soluble substances.

The Renal System at a Glance, Fourth Edition. Chris O'Callaghan. © 2017 John Wiley & Sons, Ltd. Published 2017 by John Wiley & Sons, Ltd.
Companion website: www.ataglanceseries.com/renalsystem

The principle of dialysis

If blood is separated from a suitable fluid by a semipermeable membrane, electrolytes and other substances diffuse across the membrane until equilibrium is reached. In hemodialysis, a synthetic membrane is used, whereas in peritoneal dialysis, the peritoneal membrane is used.

The principle of hemofiltration

Hemofiltration is similar to glomerular filtration. If blood is pumped at a higher hydrostatic pressure than the fluid on the other side of a membrane, then water in the blood is forced through the membrane by ultrafiltration, carrying with it dissolved electrolytes and other substances.

Practical aspects of hemodialysis

In hemodialysis, blood is pumped past one side of a semipermeable membrane while dialysate fluid is pumped past the other side in the opposite direction. The membranes are usually arranged within a cartridge as hollow fibers. The amount of fluid removed by ultrafiltration is controlled by altering the hydrostatic pressure of the blood compared with that of the dialysate fluid. The dialysate fluid is made up of the essential constituents of plasma—sodium, potassium, chloride, calcium, magnesium, glucose—and a buffer such as bicarbonate, acetate, or lactate. The blood and the dialysate equilibrate across the membrane. Plasma composition can, therefore, be controlled by altering the dialysate composition. The concentration of potassium in the dialysate is usually lower than that in the plasma to promote potassium movement out of the blood. Heparin is used in the dialysis circuit to prevent clotting. In patients at risk of bleeding, prostacyclin can be used for this, although this can cause hypotension by vasodilation.

Buffers in hemodialysis

Bicarbonate is the preferred base, but it precipitates with calcium or magnesium and must be made up just before dialysis. It is particularly useful in unstable patients and when liver disease impairs lactate or acetate metabolism. Lactate and acetate are metabolized by the liver to produce bicarbonate. However, until this occurs, the removal of bicarbonate by dialysis lowers the PCO_2 and this can inhibit ventilation, contributing to hypoxemia. Acetate is also a vasodilator and so can cause hypotension.

Dialysis access

Hemodialysis ideally requires two points of access to the circulation: one to remove blood and one to return it from the dialyzer. In the short term, this can be achieved with a large-bore dual-lumen central venous catheter. This can be tunneled through the skin to reduce the risk of infection. For long-term access, an artificial arteriovenous fistula is usually created in the arm by joining the radial or brachial artery to a vein, in a side-to-side or side-to-end manner. Over time, the fistula dilates and the high flow through it allows two large-bore needles to be placed in it for dialysis. A fistula can also be constructed by joining the artery and vein with a synthetic polytetrafluoroethylene (Goretex) graft. In renal patients, intravenous lines should always be sited on the back of the hand, rather than on the arm, to avoid damage to arm veins that may be needed later for fistula construction.

Acute complications of hemodialysis

Movement of blood out of the circulation into the dialysis circuit can cause *hypotension*. Over-aggressive initial dialysis can cause *dialysis disequilibrium*, as a result of the osmotic changes in the brain as the plasma urea falls. The effects range from nausea and headache to seizures and coma. *Headache* during dialysis can also result from the vasodilatory effect of acetate. *Itch* during or after hemodialysis may reflect the itch of chronic renal failure, exacerbated by histamine release caused by a mild allergic reaction to the dialysis membrane. Rarely, exposure of blood to the dialysis membrane can cause a more generalized allergic response, which is less likely with modern biocompatible membranes. *Cramps* on dialysis probably reflect electrolyte shifts across muscle membranes. *Hypoxemia* during dialysis may reflect hypoventilation caused by the removal of bicarbonate or pulmonary shunting as a result of vasomotor changes that are induced by substances activated by the dialysis membrane. Reducing potassium levels excessively causes *hypokalemia* and dysrhythmias. Problems in the dialysis circuit can cause *air embolism*, which should be treated by placing the patient head down on their left side with 100% oxygen.

Chronic complications of hemodialysis

The most common problems involve access and include fistula thrombosis, aneurysm formation, and infection, especially with synthetic grafts or temporary central venous access. Systemic infection can be introduced at the access site or acquired from the dialysis circuit. Transmission of blood-borne infections such as viral hepatitis and HIV is a potential hazard. Patients cannot excrete fluid between dialysis sessions so they must limit their fluid intake. If their fluid intake is excessive, the fluid is retained and can contribute to hypertension and edema. Thirst is triggered by high plasma osmolality and a major determinant of this is plasma sodium content. To reduce thirst, patients are advised to reduce their sodium intake. Reducing the sodium concentration in the dialysate can also improve the thirst. With long-term dialysis, deposition of dialysis amyloid protein containing β_2-microglobulin can cause carpal tunnel syndrome and a destructive arthropathy with cystic bone lesions. Phosphate-binding compounds that contain aluminum and aluminum contamination of dialysate fluid can cause aluminum toxicity with dementia, myoclonus, seizures, and bone disease. The condition improves with deferoxamine (desferrioxamine) treatment.

Hemodialysis in poisoning

Dialysis can be used to remove water-soluble drugs, or their metabolites following poisoning or overdose. Rapid removal may be necessary to reduce exposure of the patient to the toxic effects of a compound. Dialysis may be especially useful if renal function is impaired. Hemodialysis is fast, but in many cases, hemofiltration is also effective if dialysis is not available. Compounds that may need to be removed by renal replacement therapy include toxic alcohols (such as methanol, ethylene glycol, and isopropanol), lithium, metformin, salicylates, and rarely, sodium valproate, barbiturates, or theophylline (see also Chapter 47).

47 Peritoneal dialysis and continuous hemofiltration

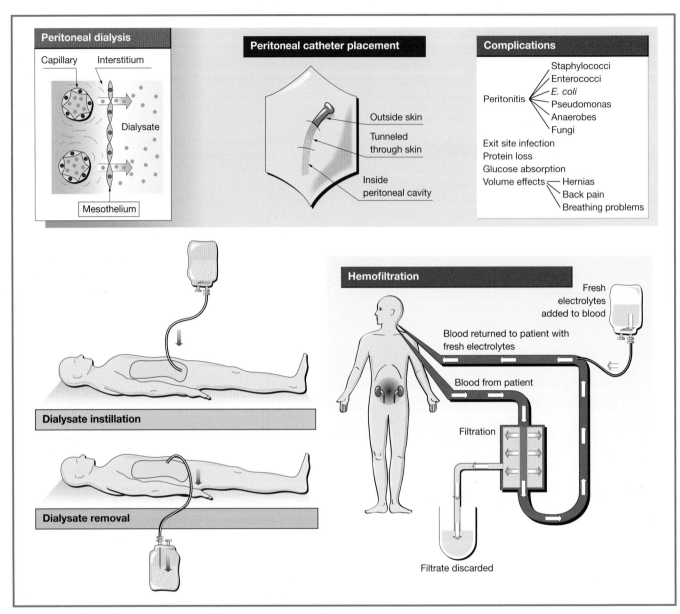

Peritoneal dialysis

In peritoneal dialysis, fluid is infused through a tube into the peritoneal cavity. Water and solutes then move across the semipermeable peritoneal membrane. The membrane consists of three layers: the mesothelium, the interstitium, and the peritoneal capillary wall. Water moves from plasma to a dialysate solution with a high glucose content by osmosis. Other molecules, such as amino acids, can be used instead of glucose in the dialysis fluid.

Solutes move with the water and also move by diffusion into the dialysis fluid. Peritoneal dialysis is slower than hemodialysis, so hypotension, hypoxia, dysrhythmias, and disequilibrium are uncommon. Peritoneal dialysis may clear some uremic toxins better than hemodialysis and is associated with less bone disease, anemia, and hypertension. However, there is a limit to the amount of dialysis that can take place, and large patients may not be able to get enough renal replacement using peritoneal dialysis.

The Renal System at a Glance, Fourth Edition. Chris O'Callaghan. © 2017 John Wiley & Sons, Ltd. Published 2017 by John Wiley & Sons, Ltd.
Companion website: www.ataglanceseries.com/renalsystem

Technical aspects of peritoneal dialysis

Soft catheters are usually tunneled through the skin and placed in the peritoneal cavity to provide permanent access to the peritoneal cavity. Formerly, semirigid catheters were used for short-term acute dialysis. Bags of sterile dialysate fluid are attached to the peritoneal catheter and drained into the peritoneal cavity by gravity. The catheter is clamped with the empty bag connected and, when the dialysis is finished, the catheter is unclamped and the fluid drained by gravity into the bag, which is then disconnected and discarded. The technique is termed **continuous ambulatory peritoneal dialysis (CAPD)** because patients can go about their normal daily activities with the fluid in the abdomen. Around four fluid "exchanges" are used each day. Typically, patients instill a fresh 2 L of dialysate every 4 h. It is common to instill a "strong" bag of high osmotic strength overnight to remove water. **Intermittent peritoneal dialysis (IPD)** is a related approach. A machine pumps fresh fluid into the peritoneal cavity every 20 min for a 12- to 48-h period. Some patients use this system every night to avoid changing bags during the day.

With both methods, any residual renal function contributes significantly to the overall efficiency of the dialysis. Peritoneal dialysis must start with small volumes and only when the catheter is secure and uninfected. Peritoneal dialysis may not be possible if abdominal surgery or sepsis has caused fibrosis, adhesions, or loss of a peritoneal surface area suitable for dialysis.

Complications of peritoneal dialysis

Infection

The major problem is infection causing peritonitis. Most infection comes from skin-derived Gram-positive staphylococci or gut-derived Gram-negative organisms, such as *Escherichia coli*, or rarely anaerobic organisms or fungi. Infection can cause fever, abdominal pain, and tenderness. Dialysate fluid is cloudy when it is removed from the abdomen and contains excess white blood cells (>100 cells/mm^3 with more than 50% neutrophils). Treatment is a few fluid exchanges to wash out the peritoneum and then normal dialysis continues, but antibiotics are added to the dialysis bags or given systemically. Usually, vancomycin is used to cover Gram-positive infection and an aminoglycoside, ciprofloxacin, or ceftazidime is used to cover Gram-negative organisms. If the infection is severe or fungal, the catheter should be removed and systemic antibiotics used. Unfortunately, repeated peritonitis can reduce the permeability of the peritoneal membrane. Infection can also occur around the catheter exit site.

Other complications

Around 5–10 g of protein is lost into the dialysate fluid each day, so protein intake must compensate for this. The use of dialysis fluid containing amino acids can be helpful. The protein loss is increased during peritonitis. A significant amount of glucose is absorbed from glucose-containing bags, and this can be troublesome for people with diabetes and may contribute to hypertriglyceridemia. Other complications include hernias, impaired ventilatory capacity, and back pain, as a result of the intra-abdominal pressure. β_2-microglobulin is better cleared by peritoneal dialysis than by hemodialysis, so dialysis amyloid is very rare. A rare but serious chronic complication is sclerosing encapsulating peritonitis (SEP) in which there is intraperitoneal fibrosis with encasement of the bowel and consequent obstructive symptoms and malnutrition.

Continuous hemofiltration

With continuous hemofiltration, venous blood is pumped at a high pressure onto a highly permeable membrane to produce large volumes of ultrafiltrate, analogous to glomerular filtration. The filtrate is then discarded and replaced by an appropriate volume of a balanced electrolyte solution, which is added back to the blood. This solution contains sodium, potassium, chloride, calcium, magnesium, and a buffer such as bicarbonate, acetate, or lactate. The great advantage of the technique over dialysis is that it is slow and continuous, which avoids the rapid solute changes of dialysis. For this reason, it is suitable for critically ill, hemodynamically unstable patients with acute renal failure or end-stage renal disease. Hemofiltration is easily performed through a dual-lumen central venous catheter. As with hemodialysis, blood is anticoagulated with heparin or prostacyclin. Continuous arteriovenous hemofiltration is an older method, which uses the patient's arterial blood pressure as the driving force for filtration.

Special related procedures

Plasma exchange

Plasma exchange removes antibodies and other large immunologically active molecules from plasma in order to treat immune-mediated diseases. Very highly permeable membranes are used to filter plasma away from the blood cells and, as in hemofiltration, the filtrate is discarded and replaced by a new solution. The replacement fluid must contain replacement electrolytes and may also contain proteins such as albumin or clotting factors. Clotting factors are removed by the process and fresh frozen plasma is usually given to reduce the risk of bleeding. Centrifugation can be used to separate plasma from blood cells in a process known as centrifugal apheresis.

Hemoperfusion

Hemoperfusion is used to remove poisons such as barbiturates, carbamazepine, and theophyllines from the blood. In hemoperfusion, blood is pumped through a cartridge containing activated charcoal which is coated with a biocompatible substance; the blood is then returned to the patient. The charcoal binds most drugs and poisons, but newer polymers and resins are being developed to bind specific substances. Columns containing specific antigens can be used to bind and remove specific antibodies against the antigen. Immunoadsorption has been used before transplantation to remove alloantibodies from patients who have antibodies against donor molecules (see also Chapter 48).

48 Renal transplantation

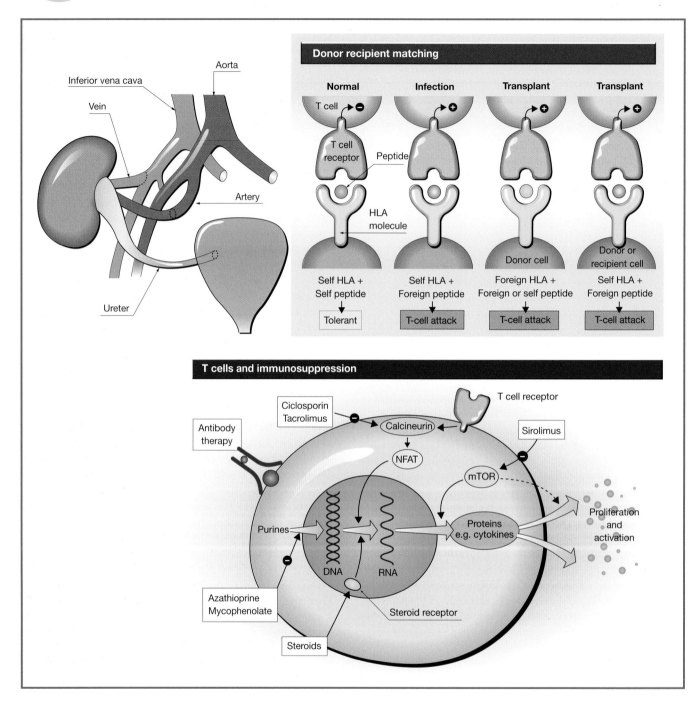

Kidneys come from live related donors or brain dead or recently deceased donors; they are implanted in the right or left iliac fossa. The renal artery is sutured to the external or internal iliac artery and the renal vein to the external iliac vein, and the ureter is implanted in the bladder wall. The immune system attacks foreign material, including transplants. Humans have many polymorphic genes, which differ between individuals, identifying transplants as foreign. To avoid immediate antibody attack, the donor and recipient must have compatible blood types.

The **human leukocyte antigens (HLAs)** are highly polymorphic proteins. HLA mismatches between the transplant organ and the recipient, particularly in HLA-A, HLA-B, or HLA-DR molecules, increase the risk of rejection and are avoided if possible. HLA molecules bind peptide fragments of protein antigens in a groove for recognition by T cells. Peptides from self-proteins are bound and recognized as self by T cells. During infection, pathogen-derived peptides are bound, which triggers an immune attack. During unmatched transplantation, T cells see foreign HLA molecules and regardless of the bound peptide,

The Renal System at a Glance, Fourth Edition. Chris O'Callaghan. © 2017 John Wiley & Sons, Ltd. Published 2017 by John Wiley & Sons, Ltd.
Companion website: www.ataglanceseries.com/renalsystem

these trigger an immune attack. Even matched HLA molecules in a transplant organ can bind peptides from other unmatched polymorphic molecules and provoke an immune attack. Other human molecules that may play a role in transplant rejection include the highly polymorphic MICA molecules, which are similar to HLA molecules.

Immunosuppression

Immunosuppression inhibits immune responses and reduces the chance of rejection, but increases the risk of infection and tumors.

Steroids such as prednisolone and methylprednisolone bind steroid receptors, inhibiting gene transcription and immunological function in T cells, macrophages, and neutrophils. Side effects include infection, peptic ulceration, osteoporosis, hypertension, hyperglycemia, obesity, mood swings, poor wound healing, cataracts, and suppression of adrenal glucocorticoid production.

Ciclosporin forms a complex with cyclophilin, which inhibits calcineurin. Calcineurin normally dephosphorylates the transcription factor NFAT, allowing it to enter the nucleus and promote expression of cytokines, especially interleukin-2 (IL-2). Ciclosporin therefore inhibits IL-2 synthesis and T-cell activation. Side effects include nephrotoxicity, hyperkalemia, hypomagnesemia, hypertension, hepatotoxicity, gum hyperplasia, and hirsutism. Acute nephrotoxicity results from renal vasoconstriction. Chronic nephrotoxicity is caused by glomerular ischemia and interstitial fibrosis. Plasma ciclosporin levels must be monitored. Drugs that induce hepatic cytochrome P450 activity lower the drug level.

Azathioprine is metabolized to 6-mercaptopurine, which inhibits purine metabolism and, therefore, nucleic acid synthesis and cell proliferation, especially in lymphocytes and neutrophils. Side effects include infection, pancreatitis, and bone marrow depression with neutropenia and sometimes, megaloblastic anemia and thrombocytopenia. Allopurinol can cause toxic 6-mercaptopurine levels by inhibiting xanthine oxidase, the enzyme that degrades it.

Mycophenolate inhibits inosine monophosphate dehydrogenase—an enzyme required for nucleic acid synthesis. Similar to azathioprine, it inhibits B- and T-cell function. Side effects include esophagitis, gastritis, and diarrhea, but usually not bone marrow suppression.

Tacrolimus binds to FKBP immunophilins to form a complex that inhibits calcineurin and so has a similar effect to ciclosporin and also causes nephrotoxicity and hypertension. Tacrolimus can cause impaired glucose tolerance or diabetes mellitus.

Sirolimus (rapamycin) also binds FKBPs to inhibit mTOR, a phospho-inositol-3 kinase. This blocks protein translation, signaling through the IL-2 receptor and the proliferation of T and B cells through the cell cycle. Proteinuria can occur with sirolimus.

Biological therapy. Polyclonal horse or rabbit antibodies against human white blood cells or monoclonal antibodies against T-cell surface molecules, such as CD3, cause white cell depletion and immunosuppression. Antibodies, such as basiliximab, block the IL-2 receptor α chain (CD25), which is required for T-cell activation and are relatively nondepleting. Rituximab is an antibody against CD20 on B cells and causes B-cell depletion, which reduces antibody-mediated rejection.

Alemtuzumab (Campath) is an antibody against CD52 on lymphocytes and causes general lymphocyte depletion. Recombinant proteins, such as belatacept (CD152 or CTLA4), that interact with regulatory molecules on lymphocytes also have immunosuppressive effects. Therapies are currently being tested that rely on promoting the development or expansion of regulatory T cells to reduce the immune response against the transplant. In some cases regulatory T cells are harvested from a patient and then expanded *in vitro* before being infused back into the patient.

Future transplantation strategies. Ideally, immunosuppression would only inhibit the immune response against the transplanted organ, leaving other responses intact. Alternatively, tolerance to the organ could be induced before transplantation.

Complications of transplantation

Early complications of transplantation

Poor renal function may indicate acute rejection, ciclosporin toxicity, or acute tubular necrosis caused by ischemia before the kidney was revascularized. Biopsy of the transplanted organ may distinguish these possibilities. Pre- and postrenal problems can also arise. **Cellular rejection** is a cell-mediated process and is treated with drugs or antibody therapy. **Vascular rejection** is more aggressive and often antibody mediated. There is usually vessel damage and plasma exchange is used to remove the antibodies. **Cytomegalovirus (CMV) infection** can cause fever, retinopathy, hepatitis, enteritis, pneumonitis, and thrombocytopenia. Treatment is with ganciclovir, foscarnet, or cidofovir.

Chronic complications of transplantation

Loss of renal function as a result of both immune and nonimmune mechanisms is termed chronic rejection. Contributing factors include immunological rejection, ciclosporin nephrotoxicity, hypertension, and recurrent disease (especially focal segmental glomerulosclerosis, membranoproliferative nephropathy, and IgA nephropathy). **Hypertension** may result from steroid use, ciclosporin-induced vasoconstriction, renin secretion by the native kidneys, or renal artery stenosis of the transplanted organ. **Hyperlipidemia** is common with steroid or ciclosporin therapy. Steroids also cause generalized **osteoporosis** and osteonecrosis of the femoral head. High parathyroid hormone (PTH) levels may cause phosphaturia requiring phosphate supplements and sometimes cause hypercalcemia. **Skin cancer** is a common late complication and the incidence is increased by sun exposure. **Post-transplant lymphoproliferative disease** is a lymphoma-like disease caused by the Epstein–Barr virus (EBV). It can occur early or late after transplantation and usually responds to a reduction in immunosuppression. **BK virus** is a polyoma virus that infects most children, but can reactivate in immunosuppressed patients causing renal impairment. The virus may be detectable in the urine and can also cause cytological changes in urinary cells. A biopsy may show polyoma virus associated nephropathy (PVAN) with inflammatory interstitial changes and tubular atrophy. Treatment is by reduction of immunosuppression, although antiviral agents such as cidofovir are sometimes used.

49 Global kidney medicine

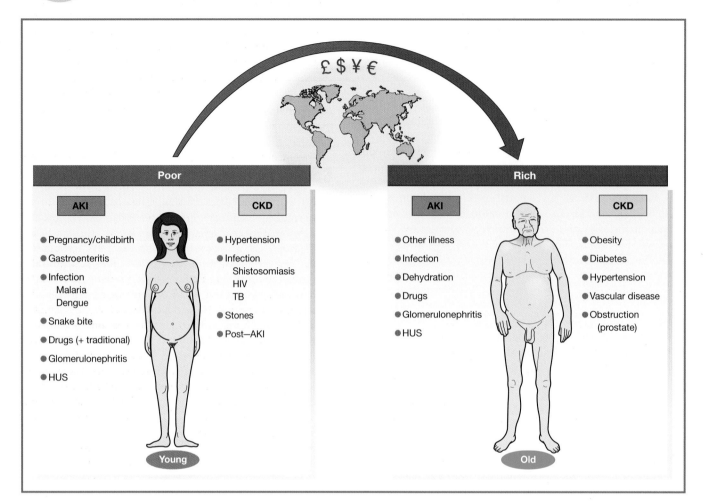

Most studies of kidney disease have focused on the richer nations in the "developed" world where kidney disease is common, but there is a huge burden of kidney disease in poorer countries too. This applies to both acute kidney injury (Chapter 41) and chronic kidney disease (Chapter 43). The prevalence of kidney diseases has probably been underestimated in countries where the resources to undertake proper monitoring are not universally available. Over time economic development is associated with a trend in poorer countries toward the pattern of kidney disease seen in richer countries.

Acute kidney injury
Richer countries

In richer countries, AKI is more common in elderly patients, typically in the context of another acute illness superimposed on co-morbidities such as pre-existing CKD, diabetes mellitus, obesity, cardiovascular disease, and in some cases nephrotoxic medication. In hospital inpatients it is usually the result of multiple factors, often including infection, drug toxicity, low blood pressure, and dehydration. The incidence of AKI is increasing with a rise in the number of elderly people in the population. Hemolytic uremic syndrome (HUS) associated with *Shigella* or *Escherichia coli* toxins remains a problem in children worldwide.

Poorer countries

The incidence of AKI in hospital is generally lower in poorer countries, but this may reflect less measurement of kidney function and so less detection of AKI or simply lack of affordable access to care where AKI can be detected and managed. In poorer countries people with AKI are generally younger than in richer countries, more likely to be female and more likely to have infection as a factor contributing to their AKI. A particular problem is that of AKI in children who have become very dehydrated, usually from severe diarrhea. Differences in access to obstetric care may influence the number of younger women who have AKI associated with pregnancy or childbirth. Important obstetric causes of AKI include infection, hemorrhage, and pre-eclampsia/eclampsia. In some poorer countries there is a notable seasonal variation in AKI which reflects changes during the year in the risk of infections such as malaria or gastroenteritis and the risk of snake bites. Snake bites are a major problem, particularly in South Asia. In poorer American nations dengue fever is an important cause of AKI. Drug causes include the standard drug causes seen in richer countries (Chapter 41) as well as those associated with plant toxins in traditional remedies.

Chronic kidney disease
Richer countries

There are many causes of CKD and some of these are common in both poor and rich countries. In richer countries, the important causes include obesity, diabetes mellitus, hypertension, cardiovascular disease with atherosclerotic disease of the renal arteries, and urinary tract obstruction, particularly in the context of prostate disease. The prevalence of CKD is rising globally because these conditions are becoming more prevalent with the lifestyle changes that are accompanying economic development of poorer countries. Globally, genetic diseases and different types of glomerulonephritis are important, but less common causes of CKD.

Poorer countries

In poorer countries a higher prevalence of AKI is likely to lead to a higher prevalence of CKD, especially if access to healthcare is limited and so management of AKI may not be optimal and may not occur at all. In addition, there are specific causes of chronic renal failure that can occur in certain contexts. Schistosomiasis, specifically infection with *Schistosoma haematobium* can cause granulomatous disease of the urinary tract that can lead to urinary tract obstruction and even cancer. HIV infection can cause glomerular disease which is generally termed HIV-associated nephropathy (HIVAN). Treatment of the HIV infection with antiviral drugs markedly improves the prognosis from HIVAN. Urinary tract tuberculosis is more common in poorer countries where the prevalence of tuberculosis is raised generally and almost always arises as a secondary consequence of lung tuberculosis. The prevalence of renal stone disease is high in hot dry countries, for example in the Middle East and this is thought to reflect relatively concentrated urine which promotes urine stone formation (Chapter 51). Drug causes include toxins in traditional or herbal remedies.

The prevalence of CKD can vary within subgroups within a country and in both Canada and Australia indigenous peoples had a higher level of CKD than people of white European ethnicity. In both the United States and Africa, there is a higher prevalence of CKD in black than white populations. These changes likely represent both genetic differences, differences in access to healthcare, and differences in lifestyle factors, which in part reflect differences in economic status.

Renal replacement therapy with dialysis or transplantation is expensive even for richer countries and so its availability tends to be very limited in poorer countries. The prognosis of people on renal replacement therapy is significantly worse than that of the rest of the population. Life expectancy is reduced to around 20–35% in dialysis patients and to around 70–80% in transplant patients.

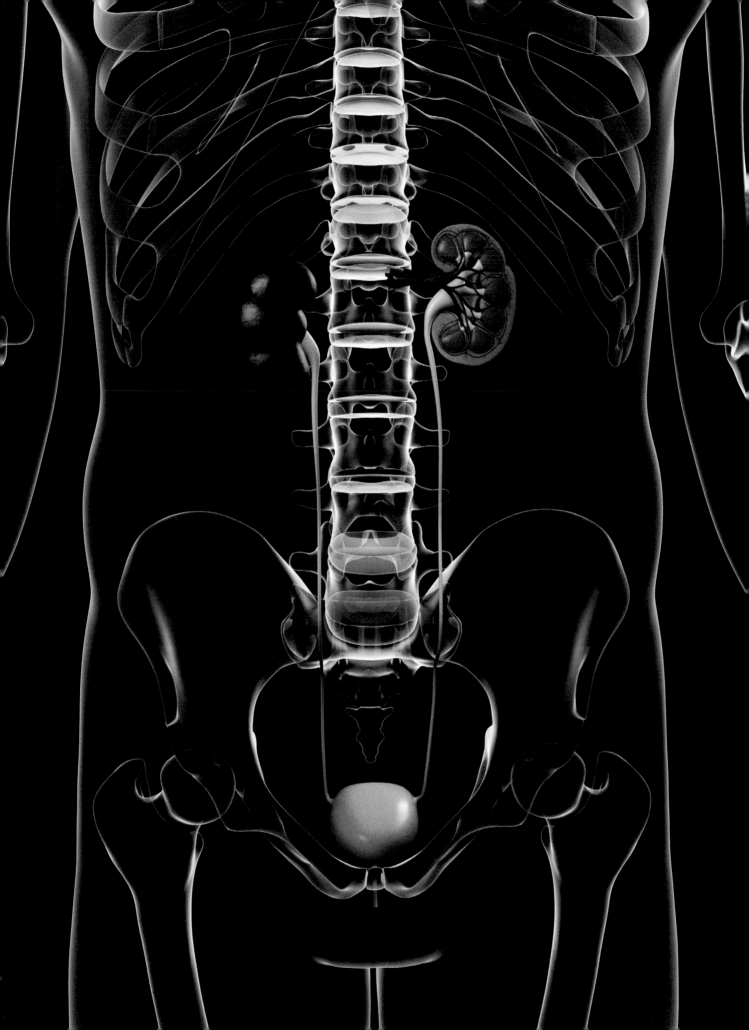

Stones, infection and cancer

Part 11

Chapters

50 Urinary tract infection 120
51 Urinary tract stones 122
52 Urinary tract cancer 124

Don't forget to visit the companion website for this book
www.ataglanceseries.com/renalsystem

50 Urinary tract infection

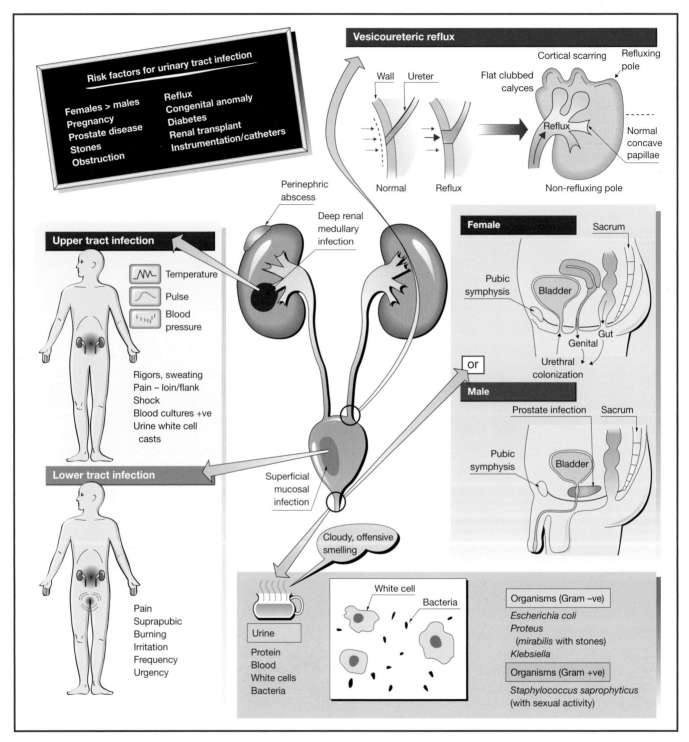

Risk factors for urinary tract infection

Females > males   Reflux
Pregnancy   Congenital anomaly
Prostate disease   Diabetes
Stones   Renal transplant
Obstruction   Instrumentation/catheters

Vesicoureteric reflux

Wall   Ureter   Cortical scarring   Refluxing pole
                           Flat clubbed calyces
                                                Reflux
Normal   Reflux   Normal concave papillae
                           Non-refluxing pole

Perinephric abscess

Deep renal medullary infection

Upper tract infection

Temperature
Pulse
Blood pressure

Rigors, sweating
Pain – loin/flank
Shock
Blood cultures +ve
Urine white cell casts

Female   Sacrum

Pubic symphysis   Bladder

                   Genital   Gut

Urethral colonization

or

Male

Prostate infection   Sacrum

Pubic symphysis   Bladder

Lower tract infection

Superficial mucosal infection

Pain
Suprapubic
Burning
Irritation
Frequency
Urgency

Cloudy, offensive smelling

Urine

Protein
Blood
White cells
Bacteria

White cell
Bacteria

Organisms (Gram –ve)
Escherichia coli
Proteus
  (*mirabilis* with stones)
Klebsiella

Organisms (Gram +ve)
Staphylococcus saprophyticus
(with sexual activity)

The Renal System at a Glance, Fourth Edition. Chris O'Callaghan. © 2017 John Wiley & Sons, Ltd. Published 2017 by John Wiley & Sons, Ltd.
Companion website: www.ataglanceseries.com/renalsystem

Infection usually enters the urinary tract through the urethra, but blood-borne infection can deposit in the kidney. Urinary tract infection is diagnosed when there are >100,000 organisms of the same bacterial species per mL of urine. White cell tubular casts suggest upper urinary tract infection.

Lower urinary tract infection is restricted to the bladder and urethra. It usually involves only the *superficial* mucosa and has no long-term effects. Upper urinary tract infection, affecting the kidney or ureters, involves the *deep* renal medullary tissue and can permanently damage the kidney.

Factors predisposing to urinary tract infection

Urinary tract infection is more common in women than in men and peaks during the child-bearing years. The short female urethra provides easy bladder access for organisms that colonize the perineum from the bowel and genital tract. During voiding, the short urethra may also cause turbulence and backflow. In women, sexual activity, especially initially or with a new partner, is associated with infection because bacteria in perineal secretions may be massaged up the urethra. Voiding before and after sexual activity reduces infection. During pregnancy, endocrine changes, especially the high progesterone level, cause dilation and reduced tone in the ureters, increasing the risk of upper tract infection (see Chapter 39). Static urine, above an obstruction or from incomplete bladder emptying, is at risk of infection. Infection can spread from a focus, such as a chronically infected prostate gland or a urinary stone (typically with *Proteus mirabilis*). Instrumentation or catheterization of the urinary tract can introduce infection, and indwelling catheters pose a continued risk of infection. Diabetes and immunosuppression, especially in renal transplant recipients, predispose to urinary infection. A single urinary infection in a woman of child-bearing age requires no investigation. In other groups, or women with recurrent or severe infection, a predisposing condition should be sought. Useful investigations include plain radiography and ultrasonography or CT scanning to exclude stones, obstruction, and anatomical anomalies. In men, the prostate must be assessed by rectal examination.

The ability to attach to urinary epithelial cells is a key virulence factor for pathogenic bacteria in the urinary tract. Some *Escherichia coli* bacteria can also invade bladder cells, which may help them to survive antibiotic courses and cause recurrent infection.

Clinical syndromes

Asymptotic bacteriuria

Routine screening detects asymptomatic bacteriuria in around 5% of women. Around 30% progress to symptomatic infection within a year. In pregnancy, this is upper tract infection, so pregnant women are screened and treated to prevent renal damage (see Chapter 39). In pregnancy, nitrofurantoin, ampicillin, cephalosporins, or nalidixic acid are used. Men with asymptomatic bacteriuria usually have prostatic disease or obstructive uropathy.

Acute, uncomplicated, lower urinary tract infection

This is common and affects mainly women of child-bearing age. The symptoms are of urethritis (burning or stinging on passing urine) and of cystitis or bladder inflammation (lower abdominal pain or discomfort, and urinary frequency and urgency). Small volumes of urine may be passed frequently and nocturia is common. The urine may be cloudy and offensive smelling. Hematuria can occur. The condition is usually self-limiting if a high urine flow is maintained by a good fluid intake. Antibiotics provide symptomatic relief and reduce the chance of chronic infection. The usual organisms are Gram-negative *E. coli*, *Klebsiella*, and *Proteus* species. *Staphylococcus saprophyticus* is also common in sexually active young women. Treatment for 1–5 days with the common antibiotics ampicillin, cephalosporins, trimethoprim, and the sulfonamides is usually adequate.

Recurrent urinary tract infection

This term refers to repeated episodes of symptomatic infection, separated by symptom-free periods, which are often simply periods of asymptomatic infection. A predisposing risk factor should be sought, although in women it is uncommon to find one. Failure to eradicate the organism from deep upper tract infection sites leads to relapse and longer courses of antibiotics may be necessary. In superficial lower tract infection, organisms are easily eradicated and relapse usually represents reinfection.

Acute pyelonephritis

Typically, there is loin pain, fever, flank tenderness, and bacteremia. Rigors can occur with malaise and vomiting. The kidney may be palpable and tender. Infection is mainly in the renal medulla with white cell infiltration around the tubules. Urine cultures and often blood cultures are positive and there may be white cell casts in the urine.

Acute complicated urinary tract infection

This term refers to infection with a predisposing risk factor such as a stone or obstruction. Antibiotics are usually only effective if the complicating factor is treated. Upper urinary tract infection in an obstructed kidney is a medical emergency and can lead rapidly to death if the obstruction is not relieved.

Vesicoureteric reflux in children

Any childhood urinary tract infection must be investigated. The major risk factor is vesicoureteric reflux caused by an abnormal entrance of the ureter into the bladder. During voiding, bladder wall contraction normally closes the ureteric orifice and the angle of the ureter in the bladder wall creates a flap valve preventing reflux. If the ureter does not pass diagonally through the bladder wall and the orifice is enlarged, voiding causes reflux up the ureter to the renal pelvis. In the renal pelvis, there may be intrarenal reflux into the medulla. The reflux usually resolves by adulthood, but most damage occurs before the age of 5 and reflux nephropathy may account for 10–15% of end-stage renal failure. The renal damage is termed chronic pyelonephritis and is diagnosed radiologically with clubbing of the renal calyces and cortical scarring. Vesicoureteric reflux is diagnosed by a micturating cystourethrogram – contrast is placed in the bladder via a suprapubic or urethral catheter, and images are taken during voiding to see if the contrast goes up the ureters. Some cases are familial.

51 Urinary tract stones

Renal tract stones

Stone type	Percentage of patients	Visible on X-ray	Risk factors in urine	Secondary causes		
● Calcium	80	Yes	$Ca^{2+}\uparrow$ $pH\uparrow$ Oxalate↑ Citrate↓ Volume↓	$Ca^{2+}\uparrow$		Malignancy Sarcoidosis Vitamin D intake
				Oxalate↑		Primary hyperoxaluria type 1 Ileal disease
				Citrate↓		Distal renal tubular acidosis
● Urate	10	No	Urate↑ $pH\downarrow$ Volume↓	With blood urate↑		Cell death Inborn metabolic defects Gout
				With blood urate normal – probenicid Acid urine – gut disease		
● Cystine	2	Weakly	Cystine↑	Cystinuria		
● Infection	5	Yes	pH↑ infection	Urea-splitting bacteria – Proteus		
● Others	3			Xanthinuria Drugs Metabolic defects		

Endemic areas of stone disease

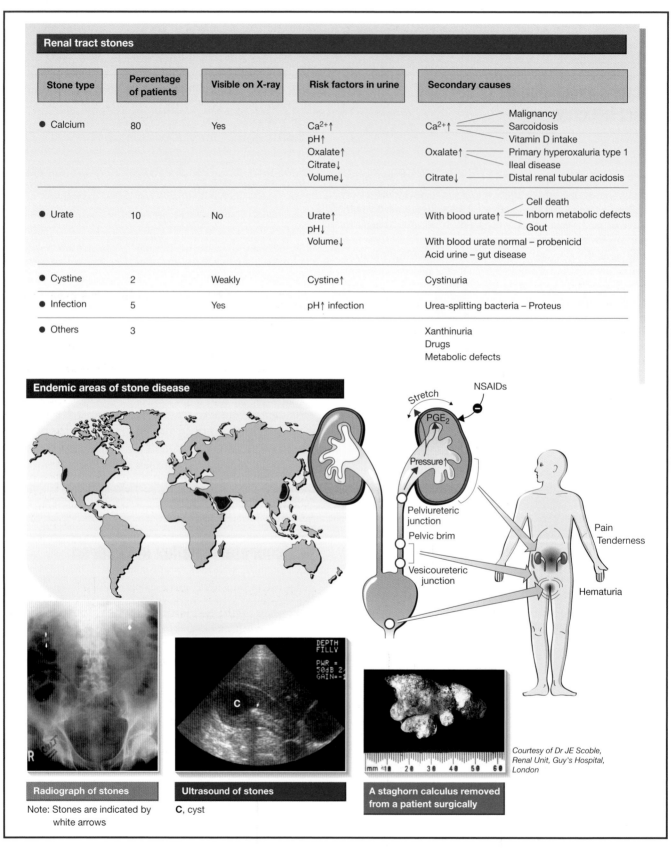

Stretch
NSAIDs
PGE$_2$
Pressure↑
Pelviureteric junction
Pelvic brim
Vesicoureteric junction

Pain
Tenderness
Hematuria

Radiograph of stones

Note: Stones are indicated by white arrows

Ultrasound of stones

C, cyst

DEPTH
FILLY
PWR =
50dB 2
GAIN=-1

Courtesy of Dr JE Scoble, Renal Unit, Guy's Hospital, London

A staghorn calculus removed from a patient surgically

The Renal System at a Glance, Fourth Edition. Chris O'Callaghan. © 2017 John Wiley & Sons, Ltd. Published 2017 by John Wiley & Sons, Ltd.
Companion website: www.ataglanceseries.com/renalsystem

Urinary stasis, infection, and indwelling catheters all promote stone formation. Stones form if stone-forming substances reach high enough concentrations to crystallize out of solution. However, debris or other crystals can promote crystal growth at lower concentrations. Urinary citrate inhibits stone formation by forming soluble complexes with calcium. Rare renal chloride channel mutations can cause stones (see Chapter 30). **Nephrocalcinosis** describes diffuse renal calcium deposition, mainly in the medulla. Causes of nephrocalcinosis include hyperparathyroidism, distal renal tubular acidosis, and medullary sponge kidney (MSK), a rare developmental disorder.

Clinical presentation

Stones can cause recurrent infection, renal impairment, or hematuria. Acute obstruction causes renal colic with intense flank pain, often radiating to the groin, and sometimes nausea, vomiting, abdominal discomfort, dysuria, renal tenderness, and hematuria. Obstruction stretches the renal capsule, causing severe pain with increased renal prostaglandin E_2 production. If there is good renal function, nonsteroidal anti-inflammatory drugs are, therefore, effective analgesics. Stones can lodge in the ureter at the pelviureteric junction, at the pelvic brim, or at the ureterovesical junction. The renal pelvis refers pain to the loin and back, the lower ureter to the testis or labium majus, and the lowest pelvic part of the ureter to the tip of the penis or perineum. Bladder stones can halt urine flow suddenly, with penile or perineal pain which may be relieved by lying down.

Calcium stones

These are the commonest type and contain calcium oxalate, calcium phosphate, or both. Predisposing factors are low urine volume, high urine calcium, high urine oxalate, and a low urine citrate level. **Hypercalciuria** occurs in 65% of patients with stones. It is usually idiopathic and associated with increased intestinal calcium absorption, obesity, and hypertension. Fluid intake should be increased and calcium, sodium, and animal protein intake decreased. Thiazides inhibit calcium excretion and potassium or citrate levels are corrected with potassium citrate. Excess calcium intake or any cause of hypercalcemia can cause hypercalciuria, especially primary hyperparathyroidism. Excess dietary sodium raises urine calcium levels by lowering proximal tubule sodium reabsorption and co-transport of calcium. Animal protein intake increases urine calcium levels. **Oxalate** is a metabolic end-product excreted in the urine. Hyperoxaluria can result from excess dietary intake, excess colonic absorption with ileal disease, or from inborn errors of metabolism. **Hypocitraturia** can be idiopathic or result from distal renal tubular acidosis, which causes excess mitochondrial metabolism of citrate.

Urate stones

Sodium urate is relatively insoluble at acid pH. Most cases are idiopathic with normal blood and urine urate levels, but often with acidic urine. Treatment involves reducing the dietary purine intake, increasing the urine volume, and urine alkalinization with sodium bicarbonate or potassium citrate. Allopurinol inhibits urate production. Secondary causes include inborn errors of purine metabolism and rapid cell turnover or death, especially during cancer chemotherapy. Good hydration and sometimes alkalinization provide prophylaxis. Acid urine is produced when there is loss of alkaline bowel contents as a result of diarrhea, an ileostomy, or laxative abuse.

Cystine stones

An autosomal recessive defect in the dibasic amino acid transporter reduces tubular cystine reabsorption, causing *cystinuria*. Cystine is relatively insoluble, especially at acid pH. Prophylaxis consists of a good fluid intake and alkalinization with sodium bicarbonate. Dimethylcysteine (D-penicillamine) cleaves cystine into soluble components.

Infection stones

These are often large staghorn calculi containing magnesium ammonium phosphate and calcium phosphate. Infection, usually with *Proteus* species, produces urease, which splits urea to produce ammonium ions. The rise in pH promotes calcium phosphate crystallization, and the ammonium crystallizes with magnesium and phosphate. Treatment involves stone removal, antibiotics, and screening for an underlying stone-forming predisposition.

Acute investigation and treatment

Plain radiography may show radio-opaque stones. Ultrasonography detects all stone types if good views are available, but CT scanning is increasingly used to image stones. Radiocontrast dye injected into the collecting system, by retrograde cannulation of the ureter or percutaneous puncture of the renal pelvis, can be used to demonstrate the site of the obstruction. Exclude urinary infection and check renal function. Stones less than 6 mm in diameter usually pass spontaneously, but stones more than 1 cm will not. Obstruction must be relieved. Stones can be removed by extracorporeal shock wave lithotripsy (ESWL), endoscopically, percutaneously, or by conventional surgery. ESWL aims shock waves at the stone through the skin, but can be complicated by bleeding and sepsis.

Investigation of patients with stones

History and clinical examination should exclude bowel disease, diarrhea, and the use of antacids and diuretics. Diet should be assessed for fluid, protein, sodium, calcium, oxalate, purine, and vitamin D intake, and a family history should be taken. Stones should be analyzed to determine their constituents. Baseline investigations include urinalysis, serum calcium, phosphate, urate, creatinine, and urea. Recurrent stone formation merits 24-h urine collections for volume, osmolality, calcium, phosphate, oxalate, citrate, urate, sodium, creatinine, pH, as well as serum sodium, potassium, chloride, and bicarbonate.

52 Urinary tract cancer

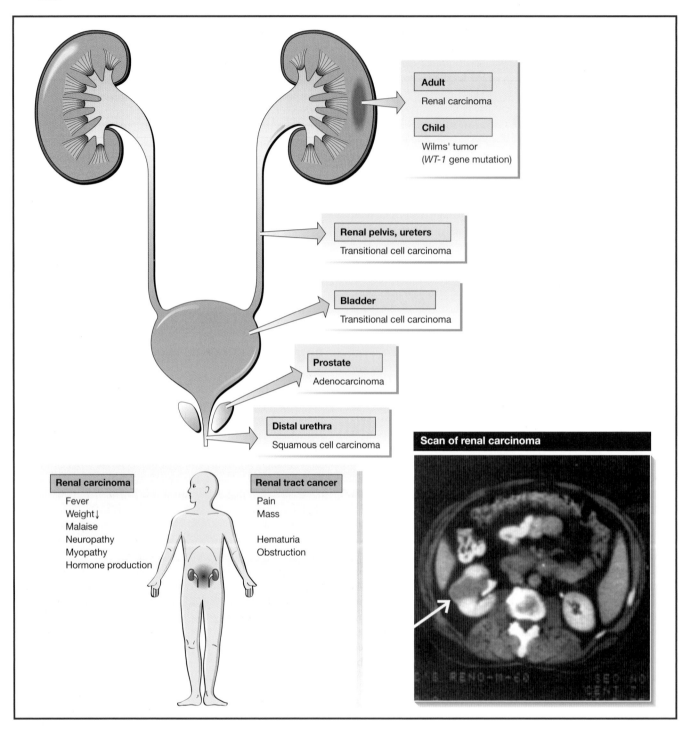

Adult
Renal carcinoma

Child
Wilms' tumor
(*WT-1* gene mutation)

Renal pelvis, ureters
Transitional cell carcinoma

Bladder
Transitional cell carcinoma

Prostate
Adenocarcinoma

Distal urethra
Squamous cell carcinoma

Renal carcinoma
Fever
Weight↓
Malaise
Neuropathy
Myopathy
Hormone production

Renal tract cancer
Pain
Mass

Hematuria
Obstruction

Scan of renal carcinoma

Tumors at different sites along the renal tract can cause hematuria or altered urinary flow.

Renal tumors in adults

Adult renal cancer usually arises in the proximal tubules and is known as renal carcinoma, renal cell carcinoma, or hypernephroma. It accounts for about 2% of adult malignancies. Most patients are over 50 years of age; the risk is increased in men and people who smoke. Most renal tumors have mutations that inactivate VHL (Chapter 9) and so activate the HIF transcription factor which promotes cancer progression. The tumor spreads locally or via the lymphatics to the renal hilum, retroperitoneum, and para-aortic nodes. It often invades the renal veins and inferior vena cava. Blockage of the right testicular vein, which drains into the inferior vena cava, causes a right-sided varicocele. The left testicular vein drains into the left renal vein, and left renal vein occlusion causes a left-sided varicocele. Metastases typically arise in the lung, liver, bones, and brain.

The usual **clinical presentation** is hematuria, but there may be loin, back, or abdominal pain. As the blood is from high in the renal tract, hematuria is usually frank and uniform throughout the stream. On examination, there may be an abdominal mass, groin, or neck lymphadenopathy, skin metastases, or a large liver or spleen. Systemic effects are common, including weight loss, night sweats, fever, anemia, nausea, malaise, polyneuritis, and myositis. Renal tumors can produce excess hormones such as erythropoietin, renin, or PTH-related protein (PTHrP) causing erythrocytosis, hypertension, or hypercalcemia, respectively. **Investigation** includes urinalysis and cytology, imaging by ultrasonography, computed tomography, or magnetic resonance imaging. Treatment is surgical removal of the tumor and often the entire kidney. Immunotherapy with interferon-α and interleukin-2 can be of benefit.

Secondary renal tumors can arise from lung or breast tumors, melanomas, or lymphomas. **Von Hippel–Lindau** (VHL) disease is an autosomal dominant condition caused by mutations in a gene on chromosome 3. It causes tumors in the kidneys, eyes, central nervous system, gonads, adrenals, and pancreas.

Wilms' tumor in children

This accounts for 8% of childhood cancers with a peak incidence at 2–3 years of age. It occurs alone or as part of a syndrome such as the WAGR syndrome (**W**ilms' tumor, **a**niridia, **g**enitourinary malformations, learning disorder/mental **r**etardation). Presentation is usually with an abdominal mass, although hematuria, pain, or fever can occur. A cure is usually achieved with nephrectomy and chemotherapy. Wilms' tumor is caused by mutations in the *WT-1* gene on chromosome 11, which encodes a transcription factor regulating gene expression (see Chapter 3).

Urothelial tumors

The renal tract is lined by transitional epithelium from the tips of the renal papillae to the proximal urethra, and by squamous epithelium in the distal urethra. Most transitional epithelial tumors arise in the bladder. Tumor in the urethra is uncommon and can be caused by spread of bladder cancers or primary urethral squamous cell carcinomas, particularly after chronic inflammation.

Bladder cancer

Bladder cancer has a peak incidence around 65 years of age. Risk factors include smoking, chronic bladder inflammation (especially from schistosomiasis infection), and exposure to industrial toxins from the dye industry. Tumors are usually transitional cell tumors, but 5% are squamous cell tumors, which usually follow chronic inflammation. Tumors are staged according to the extent of invasion through the bladder wall. There may be local spread into the pelvis, but distant metastasis is uncommon. The typical presentation is with painless hematuria. A bladder mass or obstructed kidney may be palpable. Investigation includes urine analysis and urine cytology, imaging using ultrasonography, computed tomography, magnetic resonance imaging, cystoscopy and, if necessary, examination under anesthesia. Contrast studies may show a filling defect. Sterile pyuria can occur—pus cells such as polymorphonuclear leukocytes in the absence of infection.

Superficial bladder tumors can be resected endoscopically followed by repeated cystoscopic surveillance to detect recurrence. Deeper tumors may require total cystectomy, sometimes with removal of other pelvic contents. Radiotherapy or chemotherapy may be added. Carcinoma *in situ* describes malignant change over most of the surface epithelium. It causes similar symptoms to cystitis, and is treated with intravesical chemotherapy or intravesical BCG (Bacille Calmette–Guérin) to trigger inflammation and promote tumor regression.

Prostate cancer

Prostate cancer is the third most common cancer in men. Most cancers are adenocarcinomas arising in the posterior outer zone of the prostate. They initially spread by local invasion and then involve pelvic lymph nodes, metastasizing to bone, especially the lumbar spine and pelvis, and less commonly to the lung and liver. Bone metastases are typically denser than normal bone tissue.

Presentation is usually with the symptoms of bladder outflow obstruction such as hesitancy, poor stream, terminal dribbling, frequency, nocturia, urinary retention, or obstruction. The tumor is usually hard and irregular on rectal examination. The main differential diagnosis is benign prostatic hypertrophy. Prostatic cells secrete prostate-specific antigen (PSA) and acid phosphatase, which are usually elevated in the presence of a tumor. Transrectal ultrasonography can be used to identify and biopsy tumors. Early tumors are treated with transurethral resection of the prostate (TURP) and regular follow-up. Advanced tumors may require radical prostatectomy and radiotherapy. Tumor growth may be promoted by testosterone. Hormonal therapy of metastatic disease includes orchidectomy, synthetic estrogens, androgen receptor antagonists such as cyproterone acetate or flutamide, and gonadotropin-releasing hormone analogs such as buserelin.

Case studies and questions

For each case, read the clinical section first and try to assemble some ideas about what the problem might be. This is how the clinician would have to approach the problem in real life. Then look at the investigations and see whether or not your ideas are confirmed and answer the questions. Do not look at the explanatory answers until you have answered the questions yourself.

Case 1: A 10-year-old with generalized swelling

A 10-year-old boy presented with generalized swelling. This had been present for 4 days and included swollen ankles and puffiness of the face. It started a few days after a mild cold with a runny nose. His only past medical history was of mild eczema. On examination, there were no abnormalities apart from the swelling, which included pitting edema around both ankles.

Urinalysis showed protein +++, the albumin:creatinine ratio of a spot urine was 350 mg/mmol. His serum creatinine was normal at 60 μmol/L (0.7 mg/dL), but his serum albumin was low at 20 g/L (2.0 g/dL).

- *What clinical syndrome does he have?*
- *What is the probable pathological diagnosis?*
- *What is the usual treatment?*

Case 2: A family history of hypertension and renal impairment

A 34-year-old man was noted on a routine employment examination to be hypertensive (BP 180/100). His father and his father's sister had both had hypertension and developed end-stage renal failure, and his father had received a kidney transplant. On examination there were large palpable kidneys bilaterally.

His serum creatinine was raised at 280 μmol/L (3.2 mg/dL).
What is the likely diagnosis?
What investigation would confirm the diagnosis?
What is his prognosis?

Case 3: Colicky loin pain

A 45-year-old man presented with sudden-onset, severe, right-sided loin pain. The pain was colicky in nature. On examination he was very tender in the right loin.

Urinalysis showed blood ++. A full blood count was normal. His plasma biochemistry showed a normal plasma creatinine of 101 μmol/L (1.1 mg/dL) and normal electrolytes apart from a raised calcium of 2.7 mmol/L (10.8 mg/dL). His plasma albumin level was normal at 40 g/L (4.0 g/dL).

- *What is the likely cause of the pain?*
- *What investigation would confirm the cause of the pain?*
- *Does he have a metabolic predisposition to his current problem and what might its etiology be?*

Case 4: An older man with nocturia and poor urinary flow

A 72-year-old man presented with nocturia of up to eight times a night. He also complained that the flow of his urine was poor.

He often had to wait for several minutes before the flow would start and, at the end of the stream, he experienced significant dribbling of urine. On examination he had a palpable enlarged bladder even though he had just voided.

His serum electrolytes were normal apart from a urea (blood urea nitrogen or BUN) of 20 mmol/L (56.0 mg/dL) and a creatinine of 240 μmol/L (2.7 mg/dL).

- *What is the essential part of the clinical examination that must also be performed?*
- *Why are the plasma urea and creatinine raised?*
- *What blood tests might indicate the etiology of the disease?*

Case 5: Postoperative confusion in a young woman

A 35-year-old woman became acutely confused and lethargic in hospital, 2 days after surgery for acute appendicitis. She had not been able to eat or drink since the operation. Her temperature was normal and she was well hydrated.

Her blood electrolytes showed a low sodium of 118 mmol/L, a normal potassium of 3.8 mmol/L, and a creatinine of 90 μmol/L (1.0 mg/dL).

- *What is the most likely cause of her confusion?*
- *What is the probable etiology of this disorder?*
- *How should she be treated?*

Case 6: Renal problems after vascular surgery

A 68-year-old man presented with acute severe abdominal pain. On examination he was cold, clammy, and hypotensive. Blood was taken, which showed a normal plasma creatinine of 105 μmol/L (1.2 mg/dL). He was taken immediately to the operating room, where a ruptured abdominal aortic aneurysm was identified and repaired. Two days after the operation, he was noted to be passing no urine.

His plasma creatinine was 415 μmol/L (4.7 mg/dL).

- *What are the possible causes of his acute renal failure?*
- *What investigations might help to distinguish these possibilities?*
- *What problems might require urgent renal replacement therapy?*

Case 7: Hypertension and renal impairment

A 65-year-old smoker presented with a left-sided stroke. He had weakness of the left arm and leg. On examination, he had a blood pressure of 180/95, bilateral carotid bruits, and bilateral abdominal bruits.

His plasma creatinine was elevated at 190 μmol/L (2.2 mg/dL).

- *What could explain both his hypertension and his renal impairment?*
- *What investigations might be helpful in diagnosing the cause of his hypertension?*
- *What might happen if he was given an angiotensin-converting enzyme inhibitor?*

Case 8: General malaise and itch with a pericardial rub

A 43-year-old woman presented to hospital with tiredness, itch, nausea, and general malaise. On examination, she was drowsy and pale, and had a pericardial friction rub.

Her biochemical tests showed a sodium of 142 mmol/L, a potassium of 5.1 mmol/L, a calcium of 1.7 mmol/L (6.8 mg/dL), a phosphate of 3.8 mmol/L (11.7 mg/dL), and an albumin of 37 g/L (3.7 g/dL). Her plasma urea (blood urea nitrogen or BUN) was 60 mmol/L (168 mg/dL), and her plasma creatinine was 1400 μmol/L (15.8 mg/dL). Her full blood count showed a hemoglobin level of 71 g/L, a white cell count of 6.2×10^9 cells/L (6.2×10^3 cells/μL), and a platelet count of 192×10^3/μL. A renal ultrasound scan showed two small unobstructed kidneys.

- *Does she have acute or chronic renal failure?*
- *What factors contribute to the low plasma calcium level?*
- *Is her parathyroid hormone (PTH) level most likely to be high or low?*

Case 9: A young girl with thirst and rapid breathing

A 15-year-old girl presented with a history of thirst and general malaise over 2–3 weeks. On examination, she had deep, rapid breathing and was dehydrated. Her pulse rate was 110, and her blood pressure was 90/70 lying and 70/50 standing.

Her urine showed glucose +++ and ketones +++ on dipstick analysis. Her blood tests showed plasma sodium 132 mmol/L, potassium 3.7 mmol/L, urea (BUN) 8 mmol/L (22 mg/dL), creatinine 100 μmol/L (1.1 mg/dL), and raised glucose at 56 mmol/L (1016 mg/dL). Her arterial blood gases showed a low pH of 7.05, low Pco_2 of 2.3 kPa (17.3 mm Hg) and normal Po_2 of 13.0 kPa (97.7 mm Hg).

- *What is the cause of the volume depletion?*
- *What type of acid-base disturbance does she have?*
- *What is the underlying diagnosis and how should it be treated?*

Case 10: A buried soldier with acute renal problems

A 24-year-old soldier from a bomb disposal unit was buried under rubble when a terrorist bomb exploded in a building that he was investigating. He was excavated from the rubble 18 h later by rescue workers and helicoptered to hospital. On arrival in hospital, he complained of pain in his left leg. On examination, he had multiple obvious minor injuries, but none to account for this pain. However, the muscles of his left leg and buttock were tender to palpation. He had passed only a small volume (20 mL) of dark red urine since excavation.

His blood results were sodium 140 mmol/L, potassium 7.1 mmol/L, urea (BUN) 27 mmol/L (75.6 mg/dL), creatinine 580 μmol/L (6.6 mg/dL), and creatine kinase 45,000 units/mL. His arterial pH was normal.

A cardiac monitor showed a sine wave pattern. Shortly after this was noted, he had a cardiac arrest. He was resuscitated and transferred to the intensive care unit.

- *What is the cause of his renal failure?*
- *What was the cause of his cardiac arrest?*
- *What urgent treatment does he need to prevent a further cardiac arrest?*

Case 11: Weakness and hypotension in a young man

A 24-year-old man presented with dizziness and weakness. He had a previous history of tuberculosis. On examination he was dehydrated and had a low blood pressure of 70/40. His blood results showed a plasma sodium of 125 mmol/L, potassium 6.0 mmol/L, creatinine 110 μmol/L (1.2 mg/dL), and glucose 3.0 mmol/L (54 mg/dL).

- *What is the main circulating hormone controlling renal sodium excretion and how does it act?*
- *Can deficiency of this hormone account for the raised potassium level?*
- *What is the most likely diagnosis?*

Case 12: A rash and renal problems

A 36-year-old woman presented with a cough productive of green sputum. She was treated with a course of ampicillin (a penicillin derivative). She re-presented 4 days later with a widespread rash over her arms and trunk. This was red, raised, and itchy. Her cough had improved and examination of her chest was normal.

On microscopy, her urine contained some eosinophils. Her full blood count showed a raised eosinophil level of 2×10^9 cells/L (2×10^3 cells/μL) or (20%) with a white cell count of 10×10^9 cells/L (10×10^3 cells/μL). Her plasma creatinine was 323 μmol/L (3.65 mg/dL).

- *What is the likely cause of her raised plasma creatinine?*
- *What treatment might be helpful?*
- *What steps should be taken to prevent a similar problem in the future?*

Case 13: Back pain and renal impairment

A 72-year-old retired shopkeeper presented to his general practitioner complaining of lower back pain and general tiredness. On examination he appeared pale and there was tenderness over his lower lumbar vertebrae. Blood tests showed that he had a hemoglobin of 80 g/L and a serum creatinine of 650 μmol/L (7.4 mg/dL). Immunological tests showed that he had a monoclonal band in his serum. An x-ray of his spine showed some destruction of his lumbar vertebrae.

- *What is the likely diagnosis?*
- *How can this affect the kidneys?*
- *What changes might occur in his serum calcium?*

Case 14: A sore throat and renal impairment

A 27-year-old accountant presented with a history of general malaise. He mentioned that he had recently had a sore throat, but that this had now improved. On examination, he looked well and was apyrexial, but was hypertensive, with a blood pressure of 187/94 mm Hg and mild swelling of his ankles. There were no other abnormal physical findings. His urine contained blood +++ and protein ++ on dipstick analysis. His plasma creatinine was 680 μmol/L (7.7 mg/dL). His complement levels (C3 and C4) were low, but other immunological tests were normal. A renal ultrasound was normal.

- *What is the likely diagnosis?*
- *Is there a specific treatment that should be given?*
- *What is the prognosis?*

Case 15: Hypertension in pregnancy

A 26-year-old woman was seen at a routine antenatal check at week 14 of her pregnancy and found to have a blood pressure of 120/70 mm Hg. At week 33, she was feeling tired and had noticed some swelling of her ankles. Her blood pressure had risen to 165/93 and dipstick urinalysis demonstrated protein ++. Her urine contained 1600 mg/L (160 mg/dL) of protein and 8 mmol/L (90 mg/dL) of creatinine giving her a urine protein:creatinine ratio of 200 mg/mmol (1.8 mg/mg). Her plasma urate level was elevated and her plasma creatinine was 145 μmol/L (1.6 mg/dL). Obstetric analysis indicated that her fetus was well.

- *What is the most likely diagnosis?*
- *Could she have been hypertensive before the pregnancy?*
- *Will the condition recur in future pregnancies?*

Case 16: Musculoskeletal disease and renal impairment

A 48-year-old man with a long history of ankylosing spondylitis applied for a job as a librarian. He was offered the job and attended for a pre-employment health check, where he was found to have a blood pressure of 175/90 mm Hg. Further investigations showed that he had a creatinine of 480 μmol/L (5.4 mg/dL). On dipstick analysis, his urine contained protein +++. An ultrasound scan of his kidneys showed slightly large kidneys, but no other specific abnormality. His ankylosing spondylitis had been severe, and he had damage to a number of joints including his hips and shoulders. He had ongoing joint pains and his C reactive protein (CRP) had been elevated for many years. A year previously, his creatinine had been 300 μmol/L (3.4 mg/dL). A renal biopsy was performed which showed amyloidosis.

- *Why has he developed amyloidosis?*
- *What is the likely outcome of his kidney disease?*
- *What might help to slow the deterioration of his renal disease?*

Case 17: A long illness and now renal problems

A 67-year-old woman presented with a 2-week history of sore eyes, general malaise, and joint pains affecting her knees and shoulders. On further questioning, she had not been feeling herself for nearly 6 months and had lost around 7 kg in weight over the past 3 months. Her urine contained protein + and blood ++ on dipstick analysis and red blood cell casts on microscopy. Her serum creatinine was 750 μmol/L (8.5 mg/dL). Tests for antineutrophil cytoplasmic antibodies were positive.

- *What is the likely diagnosis?*
- *What types of treatment may be useful?*
- *What are the potential side effects of drug treatments?*

Case 18: Diabetes and kidney disease

A 41-year-old woman was found to have a serum creatinine of 350 μmol/L (3.9 mg/dL) and significant proteinuria on dipstick urinalysis. One year previously, her creatinine had been 270 μmol/L (3.0 mg/dL) and 2 years previously, it had been 200 μmol/L (2.3 mg/dL). Her blood pressure was well controlled at 120/70 mm Hg and she was otherwise well. She had developed Type 1 diabetes mellitus at the age of 10 and had been on insulin since then. She had required laser treatment for diabetic retinopathy.

- *What is the most likely cause of her renal impairment?*
- *What is the likely prognosis for her kidney function?*
- *What factors influence the rate of renal deterioration in this situation?*

Case 19: A cardiac arrest and kidney disease

A 52-year-old man with known renal impairment developed severe palpitations at a football stadium. The palpitations settled, but he came to the accident and emergency department to be assessed. On arrival he appeared to have made a full recovery, but an ECG was abnormal with a wide QRS complex, and peaked T waves. Blood tests were taken, but shortly after this, he collapsed with a cardiac arrest. The cardiac monitor showed ventricular fibrillation and he was successfully cardioverted. Blood tests taken before the cardiac arrest revealed a potassium of 8.0 mmol/L (8.0 mEq/L) and a creatinine of 750 μmol/L (8.5 mg/dL).

- *What is the likely cause of the cardiac arrest?*
- *How should his high potassium level be treated?*
- *Are there any special treatments for high potassium in patients with poor kidney function?*

Case 20: Hematuria in a young man

A 26-year-old man noticed that his urine was red with blood one morning. He had been feeling a little unwell with a mild sore throat for the previous 2 days, but was otherwise fit and well. When seen by his general practitioner later that day, he was otherwise well and his blood pressure was 170/90. His urine appeared clear but contained blood +++ and protein + on dipstick testing. His serum creatinine was 180 μmol/L (2.0 mg/dL).

- *What is the most likely diagnosis?*
- *What is the natural history of this condition?*
- *Does he need any treatment at this stage?*

Case 21: An elderly man with generalized swelling and protein in his urine

An 83-year-old man presented with swollen ankles and general malaise. His blood pressure was 170/85 mm Hg and his urine contained blood + and protein ++++. Blood tests showed that his creatinine was 280 μmol/L (3.2 mg/dL), his albumin was 23 g/L (2.3 g/dL), and his total cholesterol was 12 mmol/L (462 mg/dL).

- *Does he have nephrotic syndrome?*
- *What are the likely possible causes of nephrotic syndrome in someone of his age?*
- *How can his edema be treated?*

Case 22: An otherwise well man producing no urine and coughing up blood

A 48-year-old man noticed that he had not passed urine all day, but felt well. The next day, he was short of breath and during the morning started to cough up blood. He went to hospital where his serum creatinine was found to be 350 μmol/L (4.0 mg/dL). Two weeks previously he had a routine health check, and his creatinine was 80 μmol/L (0.9 mg/dL). A chest x-ray showed diffuse shadowing throughout both his lungs and his arterial oxygen level was low.

- *Why is he coughing up blood?*
- *What are the possible diagnoses?*
- *What treatment is he likely to need?*

Answers

Case 1: A 10-year-old with generalized swelling

- This boy has nephrotic syndrome with heavy proteinuria, hypoalbuminemia, and peripheral edema causing the swelling.
- In children, the most common cause of the nephrotic syndrome is minimal change nephropathy. This typically follows an upper respiratory infection and is more common in children with atopy (allergic eczema, asthma, and hay fever).
- Minimal change nephropathy responds well to steroids. Proteinuria usually resolves completely and does not leave permanent renal damage. If the disease does relapse, ciclosporin is sometimes used to prevent further relapse.

See Chapters 33 and 35.

Case 2: A family history of hypertension and renal impairment

- The likely diagnosis is the autosomal dominant, inherited disorder of adult polycystic kidney disease. The features of this disease are hypertension, renal impairment, large kidneys, and often a family history of renal failure.
- Renal ultrasonography can easily confirm the diagnosis by demonstrating multiple cysts. Computed tomography or magnetic resonance imaging will also demonstrate the cysts.
- The prognosis is not good and progressive renal deterioration is likely. If his family members have developed end-stage renal disease, it is likely that he will as well.

See Chapter 31.

Case 3: Colicky loin pain

- This pain is typical of renal colic caused by obstruction of the right ureter by a stone. If the stone is small, it should pass spontaneously. If it is large, intervention may be necessary.
- The presence of a stone can usually be confirmed by ultrasonography and, if the stone is radio-opaque, it may be seen on plain radiographs. If kidney function is good, CT studies with intravenous contrast that is excreted into the collecting system are sometimes helpful. Occasionally, it is necessary to inject radiocontrast dye into the collecting system to identify the site of the obstruction. This can be done through percutaneous puncture of the renal pelvis or by retrograde cannulation of the ureter through the urethra.
- The patient has a raised plasma calcium concentration, and this can lead to hypercalciuria, which predisposes to calcium stone formation. There are many causes of hypercalcemia but, in an otherwise well patient, primary hyperparathyroidism is a possibility. This should be excluded by measurement of the plasma PTH level.

See Chapters 27 and 51.

Case 4: An older man with nocturia and poor urinary flow

- The patient has clear symptoms of prostatic obstruction—poor flow, nocturia, hesitancy at the beginning, and dribbling at the end of micturition. He also has a palpable bladder after micturition, suggesting that he is not emptying his bladder properly during micturition. A rectal examination is essential to determine the size of the prostate and whether it feels hard and irregular, which would suggest prostate cancer.
- The urea and creatinine are raised because glomerular filtration is reduced. The cause of this is partial obstruction of the kidney due to reduced bladder outflow, which is increasing the pressure in the urinary tract. This raised pressure is transmitted via the tubules to the glomerulus, where it inhibits glomerular filtration.
- Measurement of the prostate-specific antigen (PSA) is helpful because, if it is raised significantly, this strongly suggests prostate cancer.

See Chapters 42 and 52.

Case 5: Postoperative confusion in a young woman

- This patient has significant hyponatremia which is causing the confusion and lethargy.
- The hyponatremia is probably caused by intravenous administration of excess water in the form of 5% dextrose (glucose) solution. The dextrose is rapidly metabolized leaving only the water. Postoperatively, there is often excess vasopressin (ADH) secretion, which promotes water retention. Hyponatremia in this setting can be symptomatic and serious in a young woman.
- The treatment is fluid restriction. If no further water is administered, the kidney will gradually excrete the excess. The condition is less common if the intravenous fluid used is predominantly isotonic 0.9% sodium chloride, rather than dextrose solution.

See Chapters 13 and 14.

Case 6: Renal problems after vascular surgery

- The patient has acute renal failure with a rapid rise in plasma creatinine and a sudden fall in urine output. Several factors may contribute to postoperative renal failure. Hypotension during surgery can lead to renal ischemia and acute tubular necrosis. Renal ischemia can also arise from bleeding, inadequate volume replacement, or the undesirable hemodynamic effects of systemic infection. Postanesthetic chest infections or lung collapse can cause hypoxia, which further contributes to renal ischemia. Nephrotoxic effects of drugs, particularly aminoglycosides such as gentamicin or nonsteroidal anti-inflammatory drugs can cause renal impairment. In abdominal aortic aneurysm repair, a specific complication is damage to the renal arteries during the vascular surgery. In any abdominal surgery, damage to the ureters, although uncommon, can occur. They may be either ligated or transected.
- Renal angiography should demonstrate whether the renal arteries are intact and supplying the kidneys. Renal ultrasonography should reveal any obvious ligation or obstruction to the

ureters. If these results are normal, the presumed diagnosis is acute kidney injury caused by the multiple factors mentioned above.

• Renal replacement is indicated if there is life-threatening hyperkalemia, metabolic acidosis, pulmonary edema, or severe uremic complications, such as uremic pericarditis.

See Chapter 42.

Case 7: Hypertension and renal impairment

• The patient is a smoker who has had a stroke. The bruits indicate that he has vascular disease. The abdominal bruits are consistent with renal artery stenosis, which could cause both the hypertension and the renal impairment.

• Renal angiography is currently the best investigation for making a clear-cut diagnosis of renal artery stenosis.

• Angiotensin II levels are high in renal artery stenosis. Angiotensin-converting enzyme inhibitors or angiotensin receptor blockers can cause a rapid deterioration in glomerular filtration rate in renal artery stenosis by blocking efferent arteriole vasoconstriction caused by angiotensin II.

See Chapters 37 and 8.

Case 8: General malaise and itch with a pericardial rub

• The patient has presented with untreated chronic renal failure with symptoms and signs of the uremic syndrome, including malaise, itch, drowsiness, and evidence of pericarditis. The investigations show that both kidneys are small, consistent with chronic damage. In addition, she has anemia consistent with chronic erythropoietin deficiency. A low calcium can occur in acute or chronic renal failure, but is more characteristic of chronic renal failure.

• Factors that contribute to the hypocalcemia are a raised phosphate level caused by inadequate renal phosphate excretion and inadequate vitamin D synthesis by the failing kidney.

• PTH levels will be high. The low plasma calcium level stimulates PTH secretion (secondary hyperparathyroidism). Over time, the high PTH mobilizes calcium from bone and the plasma calcium rises. However, parathyroid cells can become autonomous and, even when calcium levels rise above normal, the PTH level may stay high (tertiary hyperparathyroidism).

See Chapters 9, 27, 44, and 45.

Case 9: A young girl with thirst and rapid breathing

• A high plasma glucose level acts as an osmotic diuretic. The glucose is filtered freely and saturates tubular glucose reabsorption. The high tubular glucose concentration has an osmotic effect, which opposes water reabsorption and causes a diuresis and volume depletion. Volume depletion is manifest as a high pulse rate and postural hypotension (blood pressure that falls substantially on standing up).

• Her pH is low so she is acidotic. The Pco_2 is also low, which in itself would cause an alkalosis. This means that the low Pco_2 represents an attempt by the body to provide some respiratory compensation for the acidosis, which is therefore a metabolic acidosis.

• The underlying diagnosis is Type 1 diabetes mellitus, and she has acute diabetic ketoacidosis. Type 1 diabetes mellitus is insulin dependent and insulin deficiency allows a high glucose level to develop, which causes the osmotic diuresis. In addition, in the absence of insulin, acidic ketones accumulate and cause a metabolic acidosis. These ketones provide a source of anions other than bicarbonate and chloride, and so the acidosis is an increased anion gap acidosis. Treatment is volume replacement with isotonic 0.9% saline solution. Insulin is given to lower plasma glucose by promoting glucose transport into cells and subsequent metabolism. Insulin also promotes metabolism of the acidic ketones. Insulin causes an intracellular movement of potassium, and it may be necessary to administer potassium to prevent hypokalemia.

See Chapters 18 and 22.

Case 10: A buried soldier with acute renal problems

• This patient has acute renal failure caused by rhabdomyolysis. His muscles were crushed by the rubble, and the pain and tenderness in his left leg and buttock are consistent with muscle injury. Damaged muscle releases potassium, creatine kinase, and myoglobin. Myoglobin colors the urine red and is a tubular toxin causing acute renal failure.

• He had life-threatening severe acute hyperkalemia. Acute hyperkalemia causes dangerous cardiac dysrhythmias. The typical ECG appearance of severe hyperkalemia is a sine wave appearance. This is a medical emergency and requires urgent treatment to prevent a cardiac arrest.

• Unfortunately, he did have a cardiac arrest. He was resuscitated, but his potassium level remains high, and he remains at risk of further cardiac arrest. He urgently requires hemodialysis or hemofiltration to remove the accumulated potassium. In the meantime, intravenous calcium can help to stabilize cardiac cell membranes, and administration of insulin can promote a temporary intracellular shift of potassium. Glucose is usually given in addition to insulin to prevent hypoglycemia. In a hyperkalemic arrest, intravenous calcium should always be administered.

See Chapters 18 and 42.

Case 11: Weakness and hypotension in a young man

• Aldosterone is the main circulating hormone controlling renal sodium excretion. Aldosterone promotes distal tubular sodium reabsorption; therefore, aldosterone deficiency causes renal sodium loss.

• Yes, aldosterone deficiency could account for the raised potassium level. In the principal cells of the distal tubule, sodium channels (ENaC) are activated by aldosterone. Influx of sodium ions into the cells can be thought of as promoting the activity of the basolateral Na+/K+ ATPase, which pumps potassium into the tubular cell. This potassium is then secreted through apical potassium channels. Deficiency of aldosterone reduces this potassium secretion, causing hyperkalemia.

• There is hyponatremia, hyperkalemia, hypoglycemia, and volume depletion. The probable diagnosis is Addison's disease with aldosterone deficiency causing low plasma sodium and high plasma potassium. Excess sodium excretion carries water with it, causing volume depletion. Damage to the adrenal cortex, which produces aldosterone, can also reduce the production of glucocorticoids. Glucocorticoids maintain blood glucose levels, so glucocorticoid deficiency can cause hypoglycemia. The adrenal cortex can be destroyed by tuberculosis infection of the adrenal glands or by autoimmune processes. Damage by recurrent tuberculosis is the most probable cause of this patient's condition.

See Chapters 12–14, 17, and 18.

Case 12: A rash and renal problems

• It is likely that this patient has an acute interstitial nephritis. She has clearly had an allergic response to the antibiotic that she was given because she has a rash and eosinophilia. The renal equivalent of this rash is an acute interstitial nephritis, which can reduce glomerular filtration causing an elevated plasma creatinine. The eosinophils in the urine are consistent with an interstitial nephritis.

• The drug thought to be the cause of the interstitial nephritis, in this case the antibiotic, must be stopped. In addition, steroid therapy, usually with oral prednisolone, is generally helpful. The prognosis is usually good and full renal recovery is usual.

• It is important that the patient knows that she has had an allergic response to a specific drug and that this is clearly recorded in her medical notes. In the future, she should not be given this drug again because the allergic effects are likely to recur. This should be explained to the patient.

See Chapter 36.

Case 13: Back pain and renal impairment

• The likely diagnosis is myeloma. This is a cancer of plasma cells, which produce antibodies. Typically, there is excess production of a single antibody. Destructive bone lesions can occur, and back pain is a recognized feature if there is damage to the vertebrae. The abnormal plasma cells proliferate in the bone marrow and normal bone marrow function can be impaired, resulting in anemia.

• Kidney damage can arise for a number of reasons. Bone disease can result in calcium release and high serum calcium levels. Hypercalcemia can lead to dehydration, which can impair renal function. Abnormal deposition of immunoglobulin protein in the renal tubules can block these tubules and cause an inflammatory response. The tubules can fill up with this protein, and this is called "cast nephropathy" because the protein can be seen to make a "cast" of the tubule. Light chain deposition can occur in which immunoglobulin light chains deposit in the renal tissue, rather than in the tubules. In addition, immunoglobulin protein can deposit as amyloid protein in the kidney, causing renal damage. It is also possible for plasma cells to directly infiltrate the kidney and impair renal function in this way.

• Serum calcium is often elevated in myeloma because of calcium release from bone.

See Chapters 27 and 34.

Case 14: A sore throat and renal impairment

• The likely diagnosis is postinfectious glomerulonephritis. This can arise following any infection, but is well documented following streptococcal throat infections. Typically, the glomerulonephritis follows the infection by around 2--3 weeks, but the interval is variable. The condition is thought to be an autoimmune disease that is somehow provoked by the infection. The clinical presentation is often of "nephritic syndrome" consisting of hypertension, fluid retention, blood and protein in the urine, and renal impairment. Complement levels may be low. The diagnosis is usually made by renal biopsy, which typically shows a proliferative glomerulonephritis.

• There is no specific treatment. Antibiotics are often given to ensure that there is no residual infection, but there is no clear evidence that this is of benefit in treating the renal disease.

• The outlook is generally good, but some patients will require dialysis and some of these will not recover renal function.

See Chapter 33.

Case 15: Hypertension in pregnancy

• The most likely diagnosis is of pre-eclampsia as she is in the third trimester of her pregnancy, has hypertension, peripheral edema, proteinuria, and increased plasma creatinine and urate levels. This could have occurred without any underlying renal disease, but occurs at an increased frequency in patients with pre-existing renal disease or hypertension.

• Although her blood pressure was in the normal range for adults at week 14, blood pressure usually falls in pregnancy because of the vasodilation that occurs. She could have been hypertensive before she became pregnant, but by week 14 the pregnancy-induced vasodilatation would have lowered her blood pressure into the normal range.

• Pre-eclampsia can recur in subsequent pregnancies, and aspirin is often used to reduce the incidence of this.

See Chapter 39.

Case 16: Musculoskeletal disease and renal impairment

• Amyloidosis occurs when there is abnormal deposition in tissues of amyloid P protein, combined with another protein. There are two types of amyloid. AL amyloid occurs in the presence of excess monoclonal antibody production, typically in myeloma, and the other protein is immunoglobulin light (L) chain. AA amyloid occurs in the presence of persistent inflammation, and the other protein is the acute phase protein serum amyloid A protein (SAA). Ankylosing spondylitis is a significant cause of persistent inflammation leading to amyloidosis. In amyloidosis, the kidneys may be enlarged due to the deposition of the abnormal protein. Proteinuria is common with amyloidosis, and this can be severe enough to cause the nephrotic syndrome.

• The likely outcome is that his kidney function will continue to deteriorate, and he will need dialysis or kidney transplantation.

• Ongoing active joint disease will continue to drive the production of amyloid protein, so controlling his ankylosing spondylitis may help to slow down his renal deterioration. In addition, his blood pressure is high, and good control of his blood pressure will also help to slow down the rate of his renal deterioration.

See Chapter 34.

Case 17: A long illness and now renal problems

• She is likely to have a form of vasculitis. Vasculitis is an autoimmune disease that can affect almost any part of the body, but commonly affects skin, eyes, joints, kidney, and lung. The most common forms of vasculitis that affect the kidney are the small vessel vasculitic illnesses, referred to as microscopic polyangiitis and Wegener's granulomatosis. These can be similar in their clinical presentation. Typically, microscopic polyangiitis is associated with cytoplasmic ANCA (cANCA) and antibodies against myeloperoxidase (MPO), and Wegener's granulomatosis is associated with perinuclear ANCA (pANCA) and antibodies against protease 3 (PR3).

• The treatment is immunosuppressive drugs, typically steroids with cyclophosphamide initially and then azathioprine or mycophenolate. Plasma exchange may be of value in some situations.

• The main side effect of treatment is infection resulting from the immunosuppression. In addition, there are multiple side effects from steroids, including gastric irritation and ulceration, acne, bruising, increased appetite and weight gain, cataracts, osteoporosis, and muscle wasting. The other drugs, such as cyclophosphamide can cause bone marrow suppression and may need to be stopped if this occurs.

See Chapter 34.

Case 18: Diabetes and kidney disease

• It is highly likely that she has diabetic nephropathy. She has had diabetes for many years and has developed diabetic eye disease. The renal deterioration has been slow and progressive.

• It is likely that her kidney function will continue to deteriorate over time and that she will eventually need dialysis or transplantation.

• There is good evidence that good diabetic control reduces the rate of renal deterioration. In addition, the use of angiotensin converting enzyme inhibitors or angiotensin receptor blockers can slow the rate of renal deterioration in diabetes. Good blood pressure control slows the rate of renal deterioration in diabetes mellitus and most renal diseases.

See Chapter 40.

Case 19: A cardiac arrest and kidney disease

• He has a very high potassium level, and this is an important cause of cardiac arrhythmias and cardiac arrest. It is likely that his high potassium has arisen because of his poor renal function. Patients with poor renal function have to avoid foods rich in potassium such as bananas.

• The first line of treatment is intravenous calcium, which can immediately provide some protection for the heart against the arrhythmias induced by the high potassium. The next step is to lower the extracellular potassium level by driving potassium into the cells. The usual way to do this is with insulin. Glucose is often given with this to avoid hypoglycemia. Ultimately, the potassium must be removed from the body. If renal function is normal, this can be done with a loop diuretic such as furosemide. It may be necessary to give intravenous fluids to prevent dehydration and to further drive urine output. It is possible to remove some potassium using ion exchange resins, which can be administered orally or rectally.

• If kidney function is poor, the kidneys will not be able to remove the potassium effectively, so diuretics will not work well. Under these circumstances, it may be necessary to use hemodialysis or hemofiltration to lower potassium levels. Usually, hemodialysis is used and can lower potassium levels more quickly.

See Chapters 16 and 18.

Case 20: Hematuria in a young man

• The most likely diagnosis is a form of glomerulonephritis known as immunoglobulin A (IgA) nephropathy. A sore throat followed within a few days by macroscopic hematuria (visible hematuria) is characteristic of IgA nephropathy. However, hematuria occurring several weeks after a sore throat can indicate

poststreptococcal glomerulonephritis. Hypertension is common, and there is often microscopic hematuria, which is detectable on dipstick testing even when the urine is visibly clear.

• IgA nephropathy can cause progressive renal deterioration resulting in end-stage renal disease and the need for dialysis or transplantation. However, some patients have very slow if any renal deterioration. A very small number of patients have an acute and severe renal deterioration.

• There is no good treatment that is specific for IgA nephropathy. However, as with most renal diseases, good blood pressure control is important and can slow the rate of renal deterioration. His blood pressure is certainly high and needs treatment. The drugs of choice in this context would be angiotensin-converting enzyme inhibitors or angiotensin receptor blockers.

See Chapter 33.

Case 21: An elderly man with generalized swelling and protein in his urine

• He has the characteristic features of nephrotic syndrome, which are heavy proteinuria, a low serum albumin, and edema. A raised cholesterol level is also typically seen in nephrotic syndrome.

• The most common cause of nephrotic syndrome in an older person is a form of glomerulonephritis known as membranous nephropathy. Other causes of nephrotic syndrome include focal segmental glomerulosclerosis, amyloidosis, and less commonly in this age, minimal change nephropathy.

• Edema in nephrotic syndrome can be difficult to control, but usually requires treatment with loop diuretics such as furosemide.

See Chapters 33 and 35.

Case 22: An otherwise well man producing no urine and coughing up blood

• He has diffuse alveolar hemorrhage and consequently has been coughing up blood. The blood in his lungs is reducing his ability to oxygenate his blood and is showing up as shadowing on the chest x-ray.

• The combination of rapid-onset renal deterioration and alveolar hemorrhage in someone who is otherwise well is typical of antiglomerular basement membrane disease (Goodpasture's syndrome). The main differential diagnosis is systemic vasculitis, but patients with vasculitis may be less well and the onset may be slower. In general, it is also important to exclude primary lung infection, which is making the patient very unwell and causing secondary renal disease.

• Antiglomerular basement membrane disease is caused by antibodies against a component of the glomerular basement membrane. The usual treatment consists of plasma exchange to remove the antibodies, steroids to reduce inflammation, and cyclophosphamide to reduce antibody production.

See Chapters 33, 34, and 42

Index

ACE inhibitors (ACEIs) 19, 35, 85, 100
  hypertension 91, 93
acetoacetic acid 53
aciclovir 100
acid excretion 47
acid–base disturbances 50–51
acid–base metabolism disorders 52–53
acid–base principles 46
acid–base regulation 48–51
  hormones, effect of 51
  liver, role of 51
  lungs, role of 51
  potassium, effect of 51
acidosis 50–51
actin 16–17
active transport 4–5
acute cortical necrosis 95
acute glomerulonephritis 78–80
acute interstitial nephritis 86–87
acute kidney injury (AKI)
  clinical aspects 102–103
  diagnosis 103
  examination 103
  global medicine 117
  investigation 103
  management 103
  pathophysiology 100–101
acute pyelonephritis 121
acute renal failure 21
acute respiratory acidosis 51
acute tubular necrosis (ATN) 95, 101
Addison's disease 30–31
adenocarcinoma 124
adenosine 15
adrenal gland 2
α-adrenergic agonists 29
β-adrenergic agonists 41
adrenomedullin 15
AE1 anion exchanger 25
afferent arteriole 2, 14, 16
afferent defect 35
aging, changes in kidney function 105
air embolism 111
albumin 3, 69
albumin:creatinine ratio 9, 85
  diabetes 97
  chronic kidney disease 105
alcoholic ketoacidosis 53
alcohols, toxic 53
aldosterone 4–5, 18, 29
  acid–base regulation 51
  bicarbonate reabsorption 54
  excess 31
  potassium metabolism 41

alemtuzumab 115
alkalosis 50–51
allantois 6
allopurinol 87
Alport's syndrome 17
amiloride 24, 38, 41
  pharmacology 71
aminoglycosides 100–101
p-aminohippuric acid (PAH) 15
ammonia production 48-49
  defective 57
amphotericin B 100
amyloidosis 83
angiotensin I 18, 28
angiotensin II 4–5, 14–15, 18–19
  acid–base regulation 51
  sodium regulation 24
  water volume regulation 28
angiotensin receptor blockers
  (ARBs) 19, 85
  hypertension 91, 93
angiotensinogen 18, 28
anion gap 53
antidiuretic hormone (ADH), see
  vasopressin
antiglomerular basement membrane
  (AGBM) antibody 79
antineutrophil cytoplasmic antibodies
  (ANCA) 11, 79
antiretroviral drugs 87
anuria 9
aquaporin (AQP) water channels 27
APOL1 gene 85, 105
aristolochic acid 87
ascites 35
aspirin poisoning 53
asymptomatic hematuria/
  proteinuria 78–80
asymptotic bacteriuria 121
atherosclerotic disease 19
autosomal dominant polycystic kidney
  disease (ADPKD) 74
azathioprine 115

Balkan nephropathy 86
Bartter's syndrome 72–73
Berger's disease 81
belatacept 115
bicarbonate (HCO_3^-) 51
bicarbonate reabsorption 48–49
biological therapy 115
BK channels 39
BK virus 115
bladder 2, 7

bladder cancer 125
β-blockers 93
blood flow through kidneys 15
blood pressure 35
blood tests 11
blood vessels 3
  loop of Henle 5
Bowman's capsule 3, 5, 14
Bowman's space 2–3, 16–17
bradykinin 14–15
buffers 46–47

calcitonin 63
calcium channel antagonists for
  hypertension 91, 93
calcium metabolism 60–61
calcium stones 123
calyx, major and minor 2–3
capillary loops 16
CaR calcium sensing receptor 61, 63
carbon dioxide (CO_2) 51
carbonic anhydrase 47
carbonic anhydrase inhibitors 71
casts in urine 8–9
catecholamines and acid–base
  regulation 51
CD2AP slit pore protein 81
central diabetes insipidus 30–31
cephalosporins 100
charge 47
chloride ions 25, 55
cholesterol emboli 19
chronic glomerulonephritis 78–80
chronic interstitial nephritis 86–87
chronic kidney disease (CKD) 104–105
  assessment 105
  global medicine 117
  management 105
chronic kidney disease (CKD),
  severe 106–107
  complications 108–109
  hematological complications 108–109
  management 109
Chronic Kidney Disease Epidemiology
  Collaboration (CKD-EPI)
  algorithm 11
chronic renal failure 21
Churg-Strauss disease 83
Chvostek's sign 64–65
ciclosporin 100, 115
cinacalcet 109
cirrhosis of liver 35
citrate 123
claudins 5

The Renal System at a Glance, Fourth Edition. Chris O'Callaghan. © 2017 John Wiley & Sons, Ltd. Published 2017 by John Wiley & Sons, Ltd.
Companion website: www.ataglanceseries.com/renalsystem

CLC-Kb/barttin channels 73
cloaca 6–7
coarctation of the aorta 91
Cockcroft–Gault algorithm 11
computed tomography (CT) imaging 11
concentration gradient 4
congenital abnormalities 6–7
congenital nephrotic syndrome 17
cortex 2
cortical nephron 14
co-transport 4–5
counter-current exchange 27
counter-transport 4–5
creatinine 10
cryoglobulinemia 83
cystatin C levels 11, 105
cystine stones 123
cystinuria 73
cytomegalovirus (CMV) 115

darbepoetin 21
dehydration 109
diabetes insipidus 31
diabetes mellitus 96–97
    histological changes 97
    treatment 97
diabetes nephropathy 96–97
dialysis 69, 110–111
    peritoneal 112–113
    poisoning 111
    practical aspects 111
dialysis disequilibrium 111
diethylenetriaminepenta-acetic acid
        (DPTA), ^{99m}Tc-labeled 15, 19
diffuse proliferative
        glomerulonephritis 81
dimercaptosuccinic acid 11
dipstick urine tests 9
disordered sodium metabolism 30–31
disordered water metabolism
        30–31
distal renal tubular acidosis 56–57
distal tube damage 87
diuretic pharmacology 70–71
    carbonic anhydrase inhibitors 71
    loop diuretics 71
    osmotic diuretics 71
    potassium-sparing collecting duct
        diuretics 71
    thiazides 71
divalent ion regulation 62–63
dopamine 14–15, 29
Doppler flow studies 11
double pelvis congenital abnormality 6
double ureter congenital abnormality 6
drug kinetics 68–69
    renal drug handling 69
drug prescription 69
dysproteinemias 83

eclampsia 95
edema 19
edema syndromes 31, 34–35
    afferent defect 35
    clinical features 35

efferent volume-conserving
        response 35
    treatment 35
efferent arteriole 2–3, 14, 16
efferent volume-conserving response 35
electrical gradient 4
electrophoresis 11
endothelin 14–15
epithelial sodium channels (ENaC) 25,
        71, 73
erythropoietin (EPO) 3–5, 20
    acute renal failure 21
    chronic renal failure 21
    hypoxic stimulation 21
    production 21
    therapy 21
erythropoietin receptor (EpoR) 20
estimated GFRs (eGFRs) 11, 105
ethylene glycol 53

Fanconi's syndrome 72–73
fatty casts 9
fenestrated endothelial cell 16
ferroportin 21
FGF23 hormone 5, 63, 107
fibromuscular dysplasia 19
filtration barrier 17
filtration fraction (FF) 15
fluid status 9
focal segmental glomerulosclerosis 81
foot processes 16–17
furosemide 24, 38, 41
    calcium excretion 61
    pharmacology 71
Gitelman's syndrome 72–73
global kidney medicine 116–117
glomerular basement membrane
        (GBM) 16–17
glomerular disease 78–79
    amyloidosis 83
    classification 79
    classification, pathological 79
    clinical syndromes 79
    cryoglobulinemia 83
    diagnosis 79
    dysproteinemias 83
    Goodpasture's syndrome 11, 79, 81, 83
    primary systemic vasculitis 83
    rheumatoid arthritis 83
    systemic lupus erythematosus
        (SLE) 11, 82–83, 86, 95
glomerular filtration 16–17
    filtration barrier 17
    regulation 17
glomerular filtration rate (GFR) 10, 15
    clearance methods 11
    estimating 11, 105
    radio-isotope methods 11
    regulation 17
    serum urea and creatinine 11
glomerular pathologies and associated
        diseases 80–81
glomerular proteinuria 85
glomerulonephritis 8–9, 102
glomerulus 2–3

cross-section 2, 16
    as filtration barrier 3
    urine formation 4
glucose 71
glucosuria 9
glycerol 71
glycyrrhizinic acid 55
Goodpasture's syndrome 11, 79,
        81, 83
Gordon syndrome 73
granular casts 8–9
granulomatosis with polyangiitis
        (GPA) 83
Guibaud–Vainsel syndrome 73

heart failure 35
hematocrit 15
hematuria 9
hemodialysis 110–111
    poisoning 111
hemofiltration 110–111
    continuous 113
hemolytic uric syndrome (HUS) 117
hemoperfusion 113
Henoch–Schönlein purpura 81
hepatorenal syndrome 35
hepcidin 21, 109
hereditary tubular transport
        disorders 72–73
high-pressure arterial stretch
        receptors 29
HIV-associated nephropathy
        (HIVAN) 81, 117
horseshoe kidneys 6
human leukocyte antigens (HLAs) 114
hyaline casts 8–9
hydrogen ion secretion 48
β-hydroxybutyric acid 53
hyperaldosteronism 30
hypercalcemia 64–65
hyperkalemia 40, 43, 51
hypermagnesemia 63
hypernatremia 30, 32–33
    clinical features 33
    treatment 33
hyperparathyroidism, tertiary 65
hyperphosphatemia 63, 65
hypertension 18–19, 90–91
    clinical evaluation 91
    complications 92–93
    pathogenesis 91
    secondary hypertension 91
    severe chronic kidney disease
        108–109
    therapy 92–93
hyperventilation 55
hypoaldosteronism 43, 57
hypocalcemia 64–65
hypokalemia 40, 42–43, 111
hypomagnesemia 63
hyponatremia 30, 32–33
    clinical features 33
    treatment 33
hypoparathyroidism 65
hypophosphatemia 63

hypospadias 6
hypotension 111
hypovolemia 55
hypoxemia 111
hypoxia inducible factor 1 (HIF1) 21, 125

imaging the kidneys 10–11
immunoglobulin A (IgA)
    nephropathy 81
immunoglobulin G4 (IgG4) disease 87
immunosuppression 115
indinavir 87, 100
infection stones 123
insulin 41, 43
integrins 16–17
intercalated cells 25, 39, 49
interlobular artery 14
intravenous urogram (IVU) 11
iron 21, 109
itching skin 109, 111

jugular venous pressure (JVP) 9
juxtaglomerular apparatus (JGA) 2, 14–15
juxtamedullary nephron 14

ketoacids 53
kidney
    anatomy, gross 3
    anatomy, micro 3
    asymmetry between right and left 3
    biochemical investigations 11
    biopsy 11
    change in function with age 105
    development 7
    drug handling 68–69
    examination 9
    functional overview 4–5
    glomerular flow rate (GFR) 10–11, 15, 17
    hormones acting on 5
    hormones produced by 5
    horseshoe kidneys 6
    imaging 10–11
    immunological investigations 11
    interstitial cells 3
    laboratory investigations 10–11
    nuclear imaging 11
    potassium channels 39
    structural overview 2–3
    tubular function 4
    ultrasound scans 10
    water regulation 26–27
kidney disease, clinical features 8–9
    examination 8
    history 8–9
    urine microscopy 8
kidney failure dialysis 110–111
    practical aspects 111

lactic acid 53
law of mass action 46
Liddle's syndrome 72–73
light chain deposition disease 83

linked transport 4–5
livedo reticularis 19
liver
    acid–base metabolism 51
    cirrhosis 35
loop diuretics, pharmacology 71
loop of Henle 2–3, 14
    acid–base regulation 48
    blood vessels 5
    potassium regulation 39
    sodium regulation 25
    urine concentration 4
    water regulation 27
low-pressure venous stretch receptors 29
lungs, acid–base metabolism 51

macula densa 2, 14
magnesium 41
magnesium disorders 62–63
magnesium metabolism 60–61
magnetic resonance imaging (MRI) 11
major calyx 2–3
mannitol 71
MDR1 ATPase transporter 69
medulla 2
medullary damage 87
membranous nephropathy 79, 81
mercaptoacetyltriglycine (MAG$_3$) 15
mesalamine 87
mesalazine 87
mesangial cells 3
mesangiocapillary
    glomerulonephritis 81
mesonephric duct 6–7
mesonephros 6
metabolic acidosis 51
    clinical features 52
metabolic alkalosis 51, 54–55
metanephros 6
methanol 53
microscopic polyangiitis (MPA) 83
minimal change nephropathy 81
minor calyx 2–3
mixed regulation disorders 30–31
modification of diet in renal disease (MDRD) algorithm 11
multiple endocrine neoplasmia (MEN) 65
mycophenolate 115
myeloma 83
myogenic reflex 15, 17
myoglobin 11

NaDC3 sodium dicarboxylate
    co-transporter 69
natriuretic peptides (NPs) 5, 15, 28–29
NBC sodium bicarbonate
    co-transporter 49
NCC sodium/chloride
    co-transporter 25, 71, 73
NCX sodium calcium exchanger 61
nephrin 3, 16–17
nephrocalcinosis 86, 122

nephrogenic diabetes insipidus 30–31, 72–73
nephron 2–3
    acid–base regulation 48
    potassium regulation 39
nephrotic syndrome 19, 78–80, 84
    clinical features 85
    treatment 85
nerves 3
NHE3 sodium hydrogen ion
    exchanger 25, 49
nitric oxide (NO) 14–15
NKCC2 co-transporter 25, 39, 49, 71, 72
nonselective proteinuria 85
nonsteroidal anti-inflammatory drugs (NSAIDs) 87, 100–101
norepinephrine 14
NPT sodium phosphate
    co-transporter 61

omeprazole 38, 87
organic anion transporter (OAT) 69, 71
organic cation transporter (OCT) 69
osmolality 26–27
    regulation 29
osmolality control disorders 31
osmoreceptors 27–28
osmosis 4–5
osmotic diuretics 71
overflow proteinuria 85
oxalate 123

panic attacks 55
papilla 2
papillary necrosis 87
paracellular movement 4–5
parathyroid hormone (PTH) 4–5, 60
    acid–base regulation 51
    calcium regulation 63
    hypoparathyroidism 65
    phosphate regulation 63
    tertiary hyperparathyroidism 65
passive diffusion 69
passive transport 5
perinephric fascia 2
perinephric fat 2
peritoneal dialysis 112–113
    complications 113
permeability 47
pH changes and potassium
    metabolism 41
pH control 52
pH and hydrogen ion concentration 46
phosphate disorders 62–63
phosphate metabolism 60–61
PLA2R phospholipase A2 receptor 79, 81
plasma exchange 113
platelet-derived growth factor (PDGF) 7
PMCA plasma membrane calcium
    ATPase 61
podocin 16–17
podocytes 16
poisoning 111

polycystic kidney disease (PKD) 74–75, 86
   clinical disease 75
   molecular pathology 75
polycystin-1 75
polycystin-2 75
polycythemia 21
polyuria 9
postinfective glomerulonephritis 81
potassium, effect on acid–base disorders 51
potassium dietary intake 39
potassium loss 35
potassium metabolism 40–41
   drugs affecting 41
   excretion control 41
   integration with sodium and volume control 41
potassium regulation 38–39
potassium-sparing collecting duct diuretics 71
pre-eclampsia 94–95
pregnancy 85, 94–95, 117
   hypertension 95
primary systemic vasculitis 83
principal cells 25, 39
proliferative glomerulopathy 81
prolyl hydroxylase domain (PHD) enzymes 21
pronephros 6
prostaglandins 5, 14–15
prostate cancer 125
prostate-specific antigen (PSA) 125
proteinuria 9, 84
   pregnancy 85
   types 84–85
proton pump inhibitors (PPIs) 87
proximal renal tubular acidosis 56–57
proximal tube damage 87
pseudohypoaldosteronism 43, 72–73
psoas muscle 3
psychogenic polydipsia 30–31
pump-leak mechanism 39
pyelonephritis 121

Q–T interval
   prolonged 65
   shortened 65

rapamycin 115
rapidly progressive glomerulonephritis 78–80
red cell casts 8–9
renal artery
   double arteries 6
   split 6
renal artery stenosis
   cholesterol emboli 19
   etiology 19
   history and examination 19
   investigation 19
   pathophysiology 18–19
   renal vein thrombosis 19
   treatment 19

renal blood flow (RBF) 15
   measurement 15
   regulation 15
renal bone disease 107
renal bruits 18–19
renal capsule 2
renal carcinoma 124
renal disease 78
renal nerves 15
renal pelvis 2
renal plasma flow (RPF) 15
renal replacement therapy 103
renal system development 6
   bladder formation 7
   congenital abnormalities 6–7
   kidney formation 7
   molecules implicated 7
   position 7
   urethra formation 7
renal transplantation 114–115
   complications 115
renal tubular acidosis 42, 56–57
renal vascular biology 14–15
renal vascular disease 18–19
   renal artery stenosis 18–19
renin 4–5, 15
   inhibitors 93
renin–angiotensin II system 15
respiratory acidosis 51, 54–55
respiratory alkalosis 51, 54–55
retinopathy 93
rhabdomyolysis 11, 102
rheumatoid arthritis 83
ROMK channels 39, 73

sacroiliac joint 3
schistosomiasis 117
scleroderma 83
secondary hypertension 91
selective proteinuria 85
sirolimus 115
Sjögren's syndrome 86
slit pores 3, 17
snake bites 117
sodium dietary intake 25
sodium regulation 24
   collecting tubules 25
   distal tubule 25
   loop of Henle 25
   nephron 25
sodium regulation by the body 28–29
sodium regulation disorders 30–31
   excess sodium excretion 31
   inadequate sodium excretion 31
sodium retention 34–35
spironolactone 35, 41
   pharmacology 71
steroids 115
stones 122–123
subepithelial deposits 81
syndrome of inappropriate diuresis (SIAD) 31, 33
syndrome of inappropriate vasopressin (ADH) secretion (SIADH) 31, 33

systemic lupus erythematosus (SLE) 11, 82–83, 86
   pregnancy 95
systemic sclerosis 86

tacrolimus 100, 115
Takayasu arteritis (TAK) 19
tenofovir 87
thiazides 24, 41
   calcium excretion 61
   pharmacology 71
thyroid hormones 41
transitional cell carcinoma 124
transplantation 114–115
   complications 115
transurethral resection of the prostate (TURP) 125
trimethoprim 43
Trousseau's sign 64–65
TRPM6 magnesium channel 61
TRPV5 calcium channel 61
tubular proteinuria 85
tubular transport hereditary disorders 72–73
tubules
   function 4
   transport processes 5
tubuloglomerular feedback 15, 17
tubulointerstitial disease 86–87

ultrasound scans of the kidneys 10
urate 95
urate stones 123
urea 11, 27
urea transporters (UTs) 27
ureter 2–3
ureteric bud 6
urethra 2
   development 7
urinary protein electrophoresis 85
urinary tract cancer 124–125
urinary tract infection 95, 120–121
   recurrent 121
urinary tract stones 122–123
urine
   appearance 9
   bedside examination 9
   casts 9
   changes in kidney disease 8
   crystals 9
   draining system 3
   electrophoresis 11
   formation 3–4
   increased frequency 9
   infectious agents 9
   microscopy 8
   osmolality 27
   pH 69
   proteinuria 9, 84–85
   red cells 9
   volume 9
   white cells 9
uromodulin (UMOD) 75, 91
urothelial tumors 125

vaptans 31, 75
vasa recta 14, 27
vascular endothelial growth factor (VEGF) 7
vasculitis 82
  primary systemic vasculitis 83
vasoactive peptides 15
vasoconstrictors 14
vasodilators 14, 93
vasopressin (antidiuretic hormone, ADH) 4–5, 14–15, 27
  potassium metabolism 41
  sodium regulation 29
  water regulation 27

vesicoureteric reflux in children 121
vitamin D 4
  calcium and phosphate regulation 63
  deficiency 64–65
  excess 65
  inhibition 5
  production 5
vitelline duct 6
von Hippel-Lindau (VHL) 21, 125

water regulation 26–27
water regulation by the body 28–29
  volume regulation 29

water regulation disorders 30–31
  diabetes insipidus 31
  psychogenic polydipsia 31
  SIAD and SIADH 31
water retention 34–35
waxy casts 8–9
Wegener's granulomatosis 83
white cell casts 8–9
Wilms' tumor 124–125
Wilms' tumor gene-1 (*WT-1*) 7
WNK mutations 73
Wolffian duct 7